INTRODUCTORY

BIOLOGICAL STATISTICS

INTRODUCTORY

BIOLOGICAL STATISTICS

RAYMOND E. HAMPTON
Central Michigan University

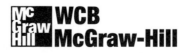

WCB
McGraw-Hill

Boston, Massachusetts   Burr Ridge, Illinios   Dubuque, Iowa
Madison, Wisconsin   New York, New York   San Francisco, California   St. Louis, Missouri

WCB/McGraw-Hill

A Division of The McGraw·Hill Companies

Book Team

Editor *Elizabeth M. Sievers*
Developmental Editor *Robin Steffek*
Production Editor *Carol M. Besler*
Publishing Services Coordinator/Design *Barbara J. Hodgson*
Visuals/Design Developmental Consultant *Donna Slade*

Vice President and General Manager *Beverly Kolz*
Vice President, Publisher *Kevin Kane*
Vice President, Director of Sales and Marketing *Virginia S. Moffat*
National Sales Manager *Douglas J. DiNardo*
Marketing Manager *Craig Johnson*
Advertising Manager *Janelle Keeffer*
Director of Production *Colleen A. Yonda*
Publishing Services Manager *Karen J. Slaght*
Permissions/Records Manager *Connie Allendorf*

President and Chief Executive Officer *G. Franklin Lewis*
Corporate Senior Vice President, President of WCB Manufacturing *Roger Meyer*
Corporate Senior Vice President and Chief Financial Officer *Robert Chesterman*

Cover and interior design by Kay Fulton

Library of Congress Catalog Card Number: 93–70484

ISBN 0–697–20209–7

Printed in the United States of America

10 9 8 7 6 5 4

Contents

3 Descriptive Statistics: Measures of Central Tendency and Dispersion   23

4 Probability Distributions   33

5 An Introduction to Statistical Inference   63

6   Inferences Concerning Two Populations   85

7   Analysis of Variance   105

Preface

The purpose of this book is to introduce upper-level undergraduates and beginning graduate students in biology to the powerful research tool of statistical analysis. Accordingly, the approach is much more applied than mathematical. It is assumed that students using this book will have math skills equivalent to a first-semester course in college algebra and will have a speaking acquaintance with probability. Perhaps of greater importance is the assumption that students using this book will have sufficient background in biology to understand why the proper design of experiments and statistical analysis are important.

This book focuses on the commonly used parametric statistical tests, their nonparametric counterparts, and the conditions under which each test is appropriate or inappropriate. The first 4 chapters cover some general concepts and probability distributions. Chapter 5 deals with statistical hypothesis testing, using inferences about a single population mean as examples. The material in this chapter is fundamental to understanding most of the material that follows and to understanding the rationale of statistical hypothesis testing and decision-making. Subsequent chapters deal with, respectively, testing hypotheses concerning two populations, analysis of variance, correlation and regression, and methods useful for nominal data and frequency counts.

My experience in discussing statistical matters with colleagues and students, in reading the research literature in my particular area of interest, and in conducting my own research is that designing an experiment or selecting the appropriate statistical test for a particular research problem or data set is sometimes a difficult decision. For this reason I have attempted to emphasize the interrelatedness of design and analysis, particularly in chapters 7 (Analysis of Variance) and 8 (Correlation and Regression), as well as the assumptions upon which the various procedures are based and the sometimes serious consequences of violating these assumptions. For this same reason, I have chosen to present nonparametric statistical tests in close juxtaposition to their more traditional parametric counterparts. Too often a parametric statistical procedure is inappropriately used in cases where a nonparametric procedure would be quite appropriate.

This book is not intended to be a compendium of all known statistical procedures, and students should be aware that there are a number of useful but less commonly used techniques that are not covered in this book. In particular, the techniques of analysis of variance are introduced, but they are not developed in depth. Rather, some of the more commonly used experimental designs and their associated computations are presented, with some examples of each, to indicate their range of usefulness.

This book is written from the perspective of a biologist who uses statistics—not from the standpoint of a professional statistician. Accordingly, my approach may be considered somewhat conservative because I emphasize that the assumptions upon which the various procedures are based should be adhered to rather closely. Thus, I have attempted to make the assumptions of the various tests clear and accessible; for instance, I have included a number of Caution boxes throughout the text to help students avoid some of the more common pitfalls in using certain statistical procedures.

With the widespread availability of computers, the actual work of doing any statistical test has become minimal. Computations that once took hours or perhaps days now take seconds or even fractions of seconds. The most time-consuming step in doing statistics with a computer is entering the data—a process that is still limited by the speed at which humans can operate. Since computers can conduct these tests much faster and much more error-free than we humans, why do we need to actually understand these tests, and in particular, the often very tedious computational steps involved? There are two reasons. First, although computers are very fast, very accurate, and have prodigious memories, they are not very smart. In fact, your pet goldfish is several orders of magnitude smarter than even the most sophisticated computer! Asked to do a totally inappropriate statistical test with a set of data, the computer will faithfully give us an answer. In fact, it could do any number of inappropriate tests with the same set of data, giving us the opportunity to reach any one of many incorrect conclusions. Computers are very good at answering questions, but they are next to worthless at asking them! That task is one that still must be done by humans. Without a basic understanding of the nature and proper use of various statistical procedures, there is a very high probability that sooner or later we will ask the computer a nonsense question and will receive a perfectly sensible looking answer. The second reason we need to understand statistical testing is simply that a computer is not always available when we need it, and even if it is, we can often more efficiently analyze small data sets and/or do certain statistical tests by hand than by using a computer. Several pocket calculators presently on the market can do a number of statistical calculations simply by having the data entered and the appropriate key pressed. You will find very frequently that such calculators are much easier to use and give results faster than computers do!

Most of the exercises at the end of each chapter may be solved with the aid of a computer, but for most of the exercises with small data sets, this would not be very efficient. Those exercises that use the larger data sets found in appendix B are excellent candidates for computer analysis and are identified by an asterisk. Since there are many statistical programs for computers in use, it is difficult to give specific instructions that would be appropriate to all of them. Most, however, and in particular the more recent ones, are reasonably user-friendly. Once one has gained an understanding of how to set up the data file for a specific computer program, the remaining steps are (usually) relatively simple. Several of the chapters include computer illustrations to solve statistical problems using MINITAB Statistical Software (MINITAB, Incorporated, 3081 Enterprise Drive, State College, PA 16801-3008), which appears to be widely used. Other programs are similar but differ somewhat in specific commands and/or file structure. Obviously, it is not possible to include specific instructions for all of the many statistical programs available.

Some of the example problems and exercises at the end of each chapter are based on imaginary but realistic data and are illustrated by the use of equally imaginary creatures. Juniper pythons, road warblers, rug rats, and the like do not exist (although they should), and one should not be unduly concerned about where such creatures are likely to be found. Many of the data sets for the examples and exercises were either suggested by "real world" experiments or were shared with me by many of my colleagues. I am grateful to the following individuals for either suggesting experimental situations for which I fabricated the data or for sharing their actual data with me: Michael Hamas, James Gillingham, Ken Zook, Pamela Keith, Jody Martin, Donna King, Herbert Lenon, John Scheide, Jennifer Kagel, Fred McCorkel, Howard Carbone, Mark Waters, Tony Ruhlman, and Dave Blaszkiewicz.

ACKNOWLEDGMENTS

I would like to thank Megan Johnson, Robin Steffek, and Carol Besler at Wm. C. Brown Publishers for their help in the development of this text. Also, I would like to acknowledge and offer a special thanks to the following reviewers for their helpful suggestions: Gary Bradley, La Sierra University, David G. Futch, San Diego State University, and John Havel, Southwest Missouri State University.

Raymond E. Hampton

Some Basic Concepts

WHAT IS STATISTICS?

Statistics may be defined as "the mathematics of the collection, organization, and interpretation of numerical data and the analysis of population characteristics by inference from sampling" and as "a collection of numerical data" (*American Heritage Dictionary,* 1st ed.). It is not inappropriate to think of statistics as the science of uncertainty; or as the science of assigning probabilities to the reliability of estimates, to the reliability of conclusions, or to the likelihood of the outcome of future events. Statistics, at its best, is another way of thinking about much of the functioning of the physical universe.

Statistics has several important uses to biologists and to anyone else who investigates variable phenomena with probabilistic rather than deterministic outcomes. One use is to provide guidance in the collection, organization, and presentation of data. Another is to determine, with a specified degree of uncertainty, if these data mean what we think they do.

CAUTION

Many of us have spent time, energy, and money conducting experiments without giving much regard to the statistical analysis that will be applied to the collected data. Very often, at the end, there is no test we can properly apply to our data because of the experimental design that was used (or because of the lack of one). Consequently, an inappropriate test is sometimes employed, either through ignorance or desperation.

With any statistical analysis there are certain assumptions about the nature of the data and about how they were collected. It is not a bad idea to think of these assumptions as rules for when a particular test may or may not be properly used. If our experimental design and data do not follow these rules, we should not use the test! Usually, but not always, violations of these assumptions invalidate any conclusions based on the test. Thus, while it is possible, computationally, to apply many different tests to the same set of data, the validity of the conclusions based on any given test depends on how well the assumptions of the test were met, not on how well the test supports the conclusion we wish to support. Any research project employs certain methods of measuring things: we measure temperature with a thermometer, pH with a pH meter, and so on. Obviously, our conclusions are no better than the least accurate of our methods. Statistical inference is one of these methods. Applying an inappropriate statistical test to our data makes no more sense than measuring temperature with a pH meter!

POPULATIONS AND SAMPLES

Statistics is generally used to make inferences about populations based on data collected from only a portion of the population. That portion is called a **sample.** A question that is properly addressed by statistical methods is: how well does the sample represent the true situation of the entire population? In statistics the term ***population*** refers to all objects of a particular kind in the universe or in some designated subdivision of the universe. One must generally take care to specify the limits of the population being investigated.

EXAMPLE 1.1   A Random Sample from a Population

The heights of a sample of 50 female students in a midwestern university were determined. The sample was selected from among all female students in the university by randomly picking their names from the student directory.   ■

We might consider this measured group to be a sample of a larger population, but what population do they represent? Is the average height of this sample a reasonable estimate of the average height of all women everywhere? What about those groups of people who tend to be unusually tall or unusually short because of genetic and/or nutritional factors? Does our sample tell us anything about them? Hardly! The only population about which we can reasonably draw conclusions is the population of female students in this university, because this is the population from which our sample was drawn. Realistically, of course, if we are willing to assume that these college women are fairly typical in stature of midwestern women in their late teens to early twenties, we could generalize our conclusion to include this larger group. Note that the key phrase here is "willing to assume." Our generalization to a larger population than the one that was sampled would be accurate only if our assumption is correct! In a purely statistical sense, we have no basis for concluding anything about the height of women who are not members of the sampled population. Imagine that, unknown to us, taller women are more likely to attend a university. Our assumption that the population sampled is representative of some larger population would be incorrect, and our generalization to the larger population would therefore be inappropriate and misleading.

Randomness

Generally, when we wish to make inferences about a population from a sample of the population, it is important that those individuals selected to make up the sample be chosen at random. **Randomness** does not imply casual, haphazard, or unplanned. Rather, it implies that each possible sample of the same size that could conceivably be drawn from this population has an equal probability of being drawn. When this is not the case—that is, when a sample is not randomly selected—the sample is said to be biased. In example 1.1, if our intention had been to conclude something about the average height of *all* women, our sample would be strongly biased because it included individuals (observations) from only one specific group of women; therefore, not all possible samples of this size from the population of all women everywhere could have been drawn. Any inference that we might make about the population based on our sample is of no value.

How does one obtain a random sample? There are a number of ways, but perhaps the most common methods involve the use of a random number table (table A.10 in appendix A is such a table). In example 1.1 we could have assigned a number to each woman in the university and then consulted the random number table to decide which individuals to include in the sample. We might do this by closing our eyes and touching the table with a pencil to select a starting number and then using consecutive numbers from left to right, right to left, top to bottom, or any other sequence. The fact that each group of numbers in this table consists of 5 digits is of no significance. This is done simply to make the table a bit easier to read. If we wish to select random numbers of three digits each, we simply read them in groups of three.

You will find it useful to consult the research literature in your particular area of interest for specific methods of selecting random samples. Essentially, individuals that constitute a random sample must be selected according to no criteria or plan whatsoever. Any method of selection that achieves this is a satisfactory method.

Independence

In addition to the requirement that members of a sample be randomly chosen, most statistical procedures assume that each sampled unit is **independent** of the others. That is to say that the choice of any one individual for inclusion in a sample does not in any way change the probability that any other individual will be chosen, or that the occurrence of some event in our sample does not in any way influence the outcome of subsequent events in our sample.

In example 1.1, 50 female students were selected at random from the student directory. Imagine that, to insure randomness, each woman's name in the entire population of university women was written on a slip of paper and placed in a box. Fifty names were then drawn from the box, which received a thorough shaking between each draw. This is a cumbersome but effective way of achieving randomness, and we may feel confident that we have selected a random sample from the population. But are the observations independent? If each name that was drawn from the box was returned to the box before the next draw (a process known as sampling with replacement), the answer is yes. On the other hand, if sampling had been without replacement (if the names drawn were not returned to the box), then the observations would not be independent. Why is this? Imagine that the entire population of women in this university consists of 1,000 individuals. On the first draw, any individual has a probability of 1/1000 (0.001000) of being selected. However, on the second draw, there are now only 999 individuals remaining in the population who may be selected, and the probability that any individual will be selected is 1/999 (0.001001). By the time the fiftieth individual is selected, the probability that any individual will be selected is 1/951 (0.001052). Thus, each time an individual is removed from a population as one of a sample and is not replaced, the probability that any of the remaining individuals will be selected increases, and the sample technically is not independent. Note, however, that the change in this probability is very small in the case outlined above, and no real harm is done to the requirement of independence. Generally, when sample size is small compared to the population size, one need not be concerned about the lack of independence that results from sampling without replacement. This is a problem, however, when the sample size is fairly large compared to the overall population size. In such a situation, sampling with replacement might be used, or one might wish to apply what is known as the finite population correction. (However, since this is an uncommon situation, the details of the finite population correction are not given here.) A not infrequent violation of the assumption of independence is when a researcher makes repeated measurements using the same experimental creature (or event) or makes repeated measurements on each of several creatures (or events).

EXAMPLE 1.2   A Sample in Which Observations Are Not Independent

An ornithologist wished to know if bluebirds prefer sunflower seeds or thistle seeds. Accordingly, two feeders were set up, one with sunflower seeds and one with thistle seeds. She observed that one bluebird visited the sunflower seed feeder 50 times and the thistle seed feeder 10 times in a certain period of time. ∎

From these observations we might be tempted to conclude that bluebirds therefore prefer sunflower seeds, and we could even conduct a statistical test (probably the chi-square test for goodness of fit) that would support our conclusion. To conduct this test, we would assume a sample size of 60, since there were 60 total visits to the feeders. In fact, the sample size is one, since we observed only one bird, and our statistical test would be meaningless! The only thing that we could logically conclude is that this one bluebird preferred sunflower seeds; we could conclude nothing about the entire population of bluebirds.

Consider a slightly more complicated version of this same situation. We tabulate visits to the feeder as before, but this time there are several birds involved. However, we do not record which bird we are counting at any particular time. It is possible—even very likely—that each bird was counted several times and that some birds were counted more often than others. Nevertheless, we then pool all of our observations to make a large sample. In this case, the sample size is not the total number of visits we recorded but the number of birds involved. Since we don't know how many different birds were involved, we don't know the sample size. This is sometimes called the "pooling fallacy," and it is almost always inappropriate. There are several correct ways of conducting this experiment—depending on the statistical test we wish to use—but the two scenarios outlined above are both incorrect because they violate the assumption of independence.

Other Types of Samples

The type of sample that we have been considering is called a simple random sample, and this is perhaps the most common type of sample used in statistical inference. It is not, however, the only type of sample that may be used. Sampling in itself is a complex subject, and it is probably wise to consult the research literature in your discipline or a statistical consultant before developing a sampling scheme for your particular research project.

C A U T I O N

A very common mistake that one encounters in the use of statistical tests, at least in the biological literature, is a lack of independence of observations. "Real life" scenarios like our bluebird example above are surprisingly common. The violation of independence of observations, when this is an assumption of the statistical test being used, is a very serious error.

KEY TERMS

independence   sample
population   statistics
randomness

EXERCISES

1.1   Using the table of random numbers (table A.10 in appendix A), select three simple random samples of 10, 20, and 30 bluegill sunfish from the data in table B.1 (in appendix B). For purposes of this exercise, we will consider the data in this table to be the entire population of interest. To take your samples, select an arbitrary starting place in the table, perhaps by closing your eyes and touching the table with a pencil. Next, record sequences of three digits as they occur, skipping any three-digit sequences that are larger than the number of observations in table B.1. When you have selected 10, 20, or 30 such random numbers, record the lengths of individual fish specified by these numbers. Use a different starting place in the random numbers table for each sample, and avoid the temptation of obtaining your sample of 30 by combining your samples of 10 and 20! Save the data so obtained for future use. Each student in the class should obtain different samples for reasons that will be apparent later.

1.2   Using the procedure in exercise 1.1, select simple random samples of 10, 20, and 30 male mosquito fish lengths from the data in table B.2.

1.3   Using the procedure in exercise 1.1, select simple random samples of 10, 20, and 30 female mosquito fish lengths from the data in table B.2.

1.4   Using the procedure in exercise 1.1, select simple random samples of 10, 20, and 30 resting pulse rates of general biology students from the data in table B.3.

1.5   Using the procedure in exercise 1.1, select simple random samples of 10, 20, and 30 reaction times of general biology students from the data in table B.3.

Data: Measurement and Presentation

VARIABLES AND DATA

Variables are characteristics that may differ from one member of a population to the next. **Data** are the values of these variables for individual members of the population.

EXAMPLE 2.1 A Continuous Variable

The heights of 5 pine trees in a certain area of forest were measured, with these results:

Tree Number	1	2	3	4	5
Height (M)	31.3	29.1	32.6	19.5	37.8

∎

In these observations tree height is a variable. A variable such as this is a **continuous variable** because it may assume any imaginable value within a certain range. Measurements of length, mass, time, temperature, concentration, and so on, are examples of continuous variables.

In other situations, we may collect data on phenomena that occur in only discrete steps or units, where intermediate values are not possible, as in example 2.2.

EXAMPLE 2.2 A Discrete Variable

In investigating the litter size of garter snakes, the following data were collected:

Snake Number	1	2	3	4	5
Litter Size	5	8	6	9	7

∎

Since fractions of baby snakes do not exist, we would never expect to obtain a measurement that is not a whole number. Variables of this kind are called **discrete variables.**

Still other variables cannot be measured on a scale in which the intervals or units have a consistent relationship to each other, yet the observations made on such variables can be ranked with respect to their relative magnitude. These are called **ranked variables.** The position of an individual in a dominance hierarchy, in which individuals may be ranked with respect to their relative position in the group, is a good example of a ranked variable. If individual A is dominant over individual B, who is in turn dominant over individual C, we may rank the individuals as A>B>C, or we may assign a number to each that indicates their relative position. Thus, A would have a rank of 3, B a rank of 2, and C a rank of 1. Note, however, that the difference between 3 and 2 need not be equal to the difference between 2 and 1. The only relationships that are expressed in ranked variables are "equal to," "greater than," or "less than."

Variables that can neither be expressed quantitatively nor ranked with respect to relative magnitude are called **attributes.** Male or female, red or white, sick or well, and so on, are examples of attributes. One may designate the class of objects to which an individual belongs, but values such as "greater than" or "less than" have no validity when applied to such attributes.

Another important class of variables often encountered in biological research is **derived variables.** Many rates are derived variables. If we measure how far a snail travels, we have measured a variable called distance. If we measure how long it moves, we have measured another variable called time. If we combine these two variables and measure how far the snail travels divided by the time of its trip, we have now measured a derived variable called velocity. Examples of derived variables are ratios, percentages, rates, and so on.

Still another type of variable that is often encountered might be called a **transformed variable.** Such a variable is the result of performing some mathematical operation on the original variable or of having a measuring device perform such an operation. An example is the measurement of pH, which, as you know, is the negative logarithm of the hydrogen-ion concentration in a solution ($pH = -\log[H^+]$). The actual variable being measured is the hydrogen-ion concentration. The transformed variable is pH.

Data are individual measurements or observations of a variable made on individual units of the population under study. Data are also sometimes called **variants** or observations. In the pine tree example, each tree is a unit of the population; height is the variable; and the height of an individual tree is a datum, variant, or observation. It is conventional to designate individual data (observations, variants) as $x_1, x_2, x_3, \ldots, x_n$, where x_1 is the first datum, x_2 the second, and x_n the nth observation in the series. When two variables are under study, one is usually designated as x and the other as y. The total number of observations of a variable in any given sample is designated as n.

CAUTION

The singular of data is **datum.**

SCALES OF MEASUREMENT

Most objects or events have at least one characteristic that is detectable and therefore measurable. Four levels, or scales, of measurement are recognized: the nominal scale, the ordinal scale, the interval scale, and the ratio scale. Each has certain distinguishing characteristics, and each may be manipulated only in certain ways.

The Nominal Scale

The **nominal scale,** sometimes called the classificatory scale, uses numbers or other symbols to classify objects or events into one of two or more mutually exclusive categories. For example, each individual in a population might be "measured" to be either a male or a female. No individual may assume an intermediate value between any two categories, nor may it be a member of more than one category. The only relationships between individuals, with respect to a variable measured on a nominal scale, are "equal" and "not equal." "Greater than" and "less than" have no meaning in the nominal scale of measurement. Attributes such as male or female, present or absent, and so on, are measured on a nominal scale.

The Ordinal (Ranking) Scale

In some instances it is possible to determine that not only are objects in different classes unlike, but also that objects in one class are either "greater than" or "less than" objects in some other class. When it is possible to determine that an object from group A is in some respect greater than or less than some object from group B, but it is not possible to determine by how much the two objects differ, we have achieved **ordinal** measurement. An example might help. Suppose we ask a group of people to describe their present emotional state as "very happy," "happy," "somewhat sad," "sad," or "very sad." In our perception of human well-being, "very happy" is greater than "happy," but how much greater? In such measurements the actual distance between any two adjacent categories ("very happy" and "happy," "sad" and "very sad") is unknown and need not be the same between all adjacent pairs of categories. Customarily, such measurements are "scored" using numerical symbols. The "smallest" item ("very sad," in this example) receives a score of 1, the next smallest ("sad") a score of 2, and so on. "Very happy," in our example, would receive a score of 5. Ranked variables are always measured on an ordinal scale.

The Interval Scale and the Ratio Scale

The **interval scale** and the **ratio scale** both have a constant and defined unit of measurement, which assigns a real number to all measurements made on these scales. Using either of these scales, not only may we specify that one object is either greater than or less than some other object, but we may specify how much greater or less. The relationship between numbers on these scales is consistent (i.e., the interval between 1 and 2 is the same as—or in some cases proportional to, in some consistent way—the difference between 3 and 4 or between any other pair of adjacent numbers). The difference between these scales is that an interval scale uses an arbitrary zero point, while a ratio scale has a true zero point. An example of the use of an interval scale is the measurement of temperature using the Celsius scale. In this scale the difference in temperature of freezing water and boiling water is arbitrarily divided into 100 equal units, each of which is called a degree, and the zero point is arbitrarily chosen as the freezing point of water. The ratio scale, on the other hand, has a true zero point, and in this case zero means there is none of the measured attribute present! Measurements of mass, length, time, velocity, and so on, utilize a ratio scale. All of the tests we will consider that are appropriate for use with interval measurements are also appropriate for use with ratio measurements and vice versa. However, when ratio or interval measurement is one of the assumptions of a particular test, it may not be used with ordinal or nominal measurements (see the caution note below). Most continuous and discrete variables are measured on an interval or ratio scale.

C A U T I O N

Many of the most commonly used statistical tests are based on the assumption (among others) that measurement is on an interval or ratio scale. When measurement is on an ordinal or nominal scale, the use of tests that assume interval or ratio measurement is always inappropriate.

Converting Data from One Scale to Another

It is not possible to convert measurements made on a nominal scale to ordinal, interval, or ratio scales, nor is it possible to convert ordinal measurements to interval or ratio scales. However, it is possible to go the other way. Data measured on interval or ratio scales may be converted to ordinal or nominal scales, and data measured on an ordinal scale may be converted to a nominal scale. Consider example 2.1, which is reproduced here:

Tree Number	1	2	3	4	5
Height (M)	31.3	29.1	32.6	19.5	37.8

Tree height is a continuous variable measured on a ratio scale. Suppose we wanted to convert these measurements to an ordinal scale for some reason (we will see later what some of these reasons might be). The shortest tree in the group is tree 4, so we assign it a rank of 1. The next tallest is tree 2, which we give a rank of 2, and so on, until we have ranked each tree with respect to the others. Tree 5, being the tallest, is given a rank of 5. Our data now look like this:

Tree Number	1	2	3	4	5
Height	3	2	4	1	5

Note that when we do this sort of conversion, we lose some information originally contained in our data. We now know only which tree is taller or shorter than which others. We do not know how much shorter or taller, nor do we know the height of any individual tree.

In subsequent chapters we will discuss a number of situations in which conversions of data from one scale to another are appropriate.

FREQUENCY DISTRIBUTIONS AND GRAPHIC PRESENTATION OF DATA

Large quantities of data, as collected, may be difficult to interpret. In this section we will consider a few basic techniques for organizing and presenting data to make them more readily understandable.

Frequency Distributions of Discrete Variables

You will recall that discrete variables may assume only certain values and that intermediate values are not possible. Example 2.3 presents a discrete variable.

EXAMPLE 2.3   Frequency Distribution of a Discrete Variable

The data in table 2.1 show the number of maple seedlings that were present in 100 one-meter-square quadrates.

Table 2.1   *Maple Seedlings per One-Meter-Square Quadrate*

0	1	0	2	0	0	1	2	1	1	3	4
0	1	2	5	1	0	2	1	1	2	1	3
1	2	3	4	3	4	2	1	0	5	5	2
0	0	2	0	1	0	0	0	2	0	1	0
1	3	4	2	1	0	0	1	0	1	1	0
2	3	5	0	0	0	1	2	3	4	3	4
3	3	0	2	0	4	5	0	0	0	1	1
0	1	0	0	1	0	1	0	0	1	1	2
0	1	0	1								

Data from M. Hamas   ■

Clearly data in this form are rather difficult to interpret. From glancing through the numbers it would seem that the quadrates contained about 2 or 3 plants each, except that many contained no plants at all. As an initial step in analyzing data, it is frequently advantageous to group the data into a **frequency distribution.** In this case we would determine how many quadrates contained 0 plants, how many contained 1 plant, how many contained 2 plants, and so on. We would then tabulate the results in the manner shown in table 2.2. This arrangement makes the data much easier to deal with. We can see at a glance that 35 quadrates contained 0 seedlings, 28 contained only 1, and so on. A frequency distribution is often represented in the form of a **bar graph,** which makes the information it contains even more immediately accessible. Figure 2.1 is such a bar graph, constructed from the frequency distribution in table 2.2.

Table 2.2   *Maple Seedlings per Quadrate*

Number of Plants/Quadrate	*Frequency*
0	35
1	28
2	15
3	10
4	7
5	5

In effect we are plotting a variable along the x-axis (in this case, the number of plants per quadrate) against the number of times that variable occurred (its frequency) on the y-axis. Graphs of frequency distributions are often called **histograms** if the variable graphed is continuous, and bar graphs if the variable is discontinuous (as in this case), and we will have many occasions to make use of them. Note that the bars in figure 2.1 representing the various **frequencies** do not touch each other. This is because a discrete variable is involved, and intermediate values are not possible. Discrete variables are conventionally plotted this way.

Frequency Distributions of Continuous Variables

You will recall that continuous variables may assume any imaginable value between certain limits. Accordingly, their graphic and tabular presentations are somewhat different from those of discrete variables.

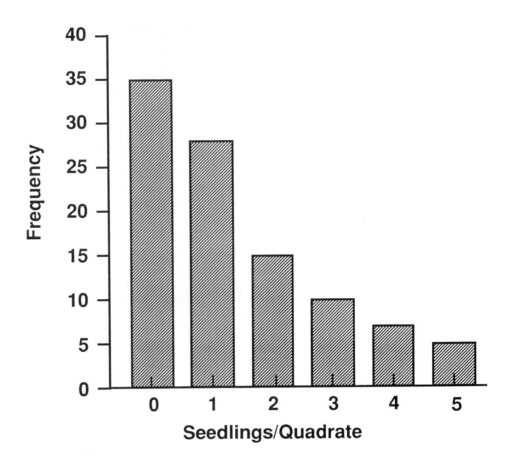

Figure 2.1
Maple seedlings per quadrate
(an example of a bar graph).

EXAMPLE 2.4   Frequency Distribution of a Continuous Variable

A simple random sample of 172 adult male mosquito fish was collected from a large population, and the total length of each fish was measured to the nearest millimeter. These data are shown in table 2.3.

Table 2.3   Total Lengths of 172 Male Mosquito Fish
(in millimeters)

30	22	23	28	19	22	21	23	22	24	20	23
17	22	24	20	20	23	20	18	21	25	22	29
19	22	21	20	20	23	22	18	22	21	22	21
22	24	17	22	23	21	21	19	24	20	23	21
19	22	22	21	23	20	21	20	20	23	20	21
22	20	20	24	24	24	18	19	21	21	19	21
24	19	22	23	24	28	22	24	21	20	24	24
23	23	22	22	21	21	22	20	21	24	22	23
23	21	25	25	24	25	23	23	22	20	21	24
19	22	23	22	24	24	19	20	24	24	21	22
22	23	25	22	20	20	24	20	23	22	21	22
22	21	20	21	24	20	24	21	21	22	19	21
19	22	23	22	22	22	20	23	22	22	24	20
22	21	23	23	20	21	21	20	21	22	26	24
19	22	20	20								

■

Once again, inspection of the data in this form makes interpretation difficult. Length is a continuous variable measured on a ratio scale, and the information contained in a frequency distribution of such a variable is somewhat different from that contained in a frequency distribution of a discrete variable. A continuous variable may assume any value within a certain range, while a discrete variable may not. Thus, when constructing a frequency distribution of a continuous variable, it is customary to group measurements into classes containing only individuals that fall within a certain range of the variable under consideration. For example, we might group all of the male mosquito fish lengths in table 2.3 that measured 17 mm and 18 mm into one class, those that measured 19 mm and 20 mm into another, and so on. Keep in mind that measurement was to the nearest millimeter, so that, in effect, 17 mm really includes individuals from 16.5 mm to 17.5 mm, and so on. Thus, our 17 mm to 18 mm class actually includes individuals from 16.5 mm to 18.5 mm (a range of 2 mm) and our 19 mm to 20 mm class includes individuals from 18.5 mm to 20.5 mm (also a range of 2 mm). In this case we are using a class interval of 2 mm. The choice of class interval is somewhat arbitrary and depends to some extent on the number of data and on the range of the measurements. Too many classes tend to be confusing, while too few convey too little information. Trial and error is not a bad way of arriving at a satisfactory class interval! Once a class interval is chosen, a value halfway between the smaller and the larger limit of each class is designated as the class mark. For example, in the 16.5 mm to 18.5 mm class above, 17.5 mm is the class mark. The class mark for the 18.5 mm to 20.5 mm class interval is 19.5 mm, and so on.

Table 2.4 is a frequency distribution of the data in table 2.3, using a class interval of 2 mm. The smallest fish in the sample was 17 mm (actually 16.5 mm to 17.5 mm), which tells us that the first class includes all individuals that were between 16.5 mm and 18.5 mm. In other words, it includes all of those individuals that had a measured length of 17 mm or 18 mm. The second class includes individuals between 18.5 mm and 20.5 mm, and so on.

Table 2.4   Total Length of Male Mosquito Fish (in millimeters)

Measured Length	Implied Length	Class Mark	Frequency
17–18	16.5–18.5	17.5	5
19–20	18.5–20.5	19.5	40
21–22	20.5–22.5	21.5	70
23–24	22.5–24.5	23.5	47
25–26	24.5–26.5	25.5	6
27–28	26.5–28.5	27.5	2
29–30	28.5–30.5	29.5	2

Figure 2.2 is a histogram of the frequency distribution given in table 2.4. Note that in the distribution in table 2.4 and in the histogram in figure 2.2 there is no "space" between classes. This reflects the basic nature of a continuous variable. In some instances the classes used to construct a histogram are not equal. In such cases the width of the bars should be proportional to the class interval being depicted.

There is a second common way to graph distributions of a continuous variable. Rather than using bars, points are plotted on a graph with the class marks on the *x*-axis and the frequency on the *y*-axis. Such a graph is called a **frequency polygon,** and an example is shown in figure 2.3, again using the data from tables 2.3 and 2.4. With small class intervals and large sample sizes,

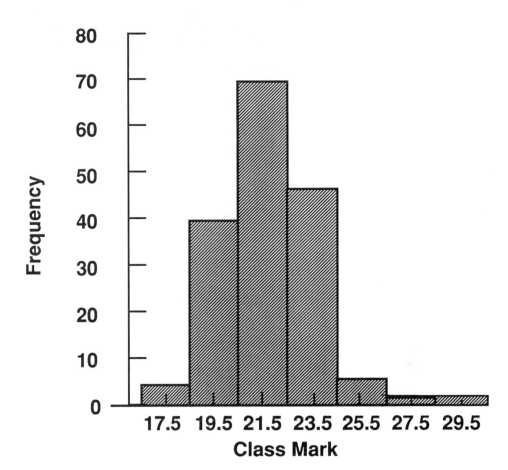

Figure 2.2
Frequency distribution of male
mosquito fish length (an
example of a histogram).

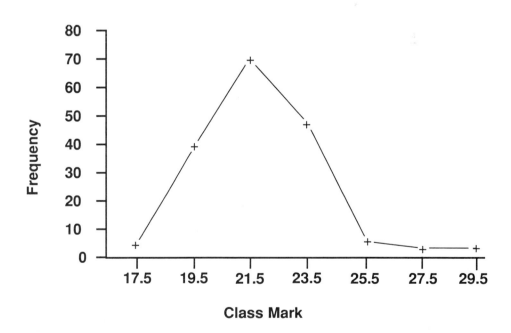

Figure 2.3
Frequency distribution of male
mosquito fish length (an
example of a frequency
polygon).

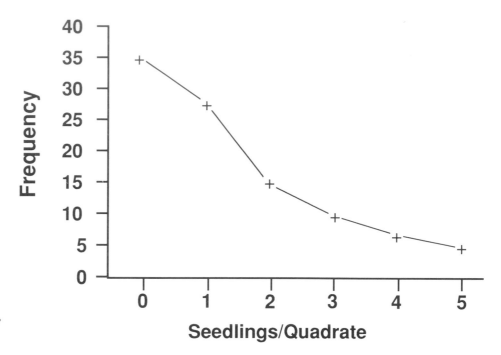

Figure 2.4
Maple seedlings per quadrate
(an example of the incorrect use
of a continuous line graph).

or for approximations with smaller sample sizes, frequency polygons are quite acceptable. Note that frequency polygons cannot be properly used to show the frequency distribution of a discrete variable since the line "connecting the dots" indicates that the variable is continuous.

C A U T I O N

It is not uncommon to see graphs of discrete variables presented as continuous line graphs rather than as bar graphs. Refer to figure 2.1, which is the bar graph for the maple-seedlings-per-quadrate example. This is clearly a discrete variable, and the bar graph in figure 2.1 is the proper way to present such data graphically. However, the data could be plotted as shown in figure 2.4, with the dots corresponding to the bars in figure 2.1. Note that the dots are connected by a solid line. What a graph like that in figure 2.4 indicates is that any value of the variable (number of seedlings in a quadrate) between 0 and 5 can occur and that any frequency between 0 and 35 can occur. If we interpolate roughly from this graph we might conclude that we observed about 22.3 quadrates with 1.4 maple seedlings! Line graphs are for continuous variables, in which the variable can assume any intermediate value. Bar graphs are for discrete variables, in which intermediated values are not possible.

COMPUTER SUPPLEMENT

Most statistical programs for computers have some graphing capabilities. MINITAB is capable of producing several types of graphic representations of frequency distributions. Figure 2.5 is a histogram generated by the MINITAB program of the data from example 2.4.

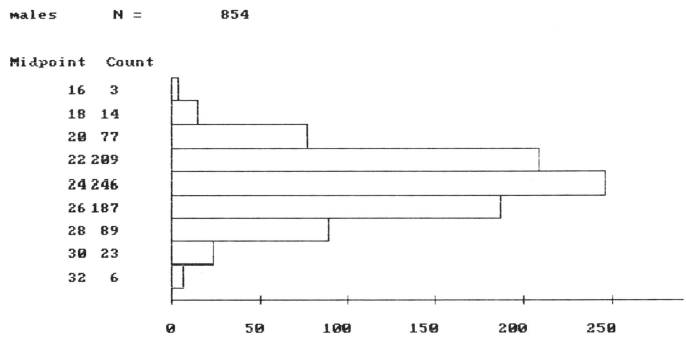

Figure 2.5
MINITAB-generated histogram of male mosquito fish length. Compare with figure 2.2.

KEY TERMS

attribute	histogram
bar graph	interval scale
continuous variable	nominal scale
data (datum)	ordinal scale
derived variable	ranked variable
discrete variable	ratio scale
frequency	transformed variable
frequency distribution	variable
frequency polygon	variant

(Exercises preceded by an asterisk are suitable for computer solution.)

2.1 Below are the heights (in centimeters) of a sample of 148 male humans.

187	171	181	180	178	171	174	177	172	178	182
187	176	179	190	185	192	184	182	178	187	173
185	184	184	183	185	197	202	181	181	191	178
187	185	186	174	174	182	195	182	180	182	182
179	183	178	185	178	190	180	175	169	176	182
185	179	180	187	178	170	181	200	161	181	173
178	182	181	181	181	172	185	188	188	177	176
173	174	176	189	180	182	188	184	179	177	177
183	196	184	173	180	180	180	184	175	176	186
187	182	187	174	178	191	182	174	178	191	178
173	183	191	191	180	187	184	177	186	194	185
189	193	189	192	189	181	177	176	190	173	179
180	184	176	180	178	171	182	173	184	193	182
185	178	190	190	183						

2.1a What is the scale of measurement by which this variable was measured?

2.1b Is this a discrete or continuous variable?

2.1c Construct a frequency distribution table and a histogram of these data. A class interval of 2 cm is suggested.

2.2 Given below are the lengths (in millimeters) of a sample of 100 largemouth bass.

210	325	285	402	350	240	409	330	295	325
241	383	361	355	200	432	130	114	170	135
371	307	207	175	177	261	166	376	216	152
347	322	387	233	284	394	297	321	281	66
90	115	250	201	175	320	370	312	370	320
175	201	250	115	95	70	289	312	322	258
188	192	350	200	199	180	190	180	200	200
349	192	189	260	320	432	456	331	418	357
304	316	336	368	415	370	336	315	305	420
310	397	193	394	199	338	296	312	269	203

2.2a What is the scale of measurement by which this variable was measured?

2.2b Is this a continuous or discrete variable?

2.2c Construct a frequency distribution table and histogram of these data.

2.3 An ecology class determined the number of ant lion pits in a sample of 100 randomly selected one-meter-square quadrates. The results were as follows.

Pits/Quadrate (x)	Number of Quadrates Containing x Pits(Frequency)
0	5
1	15
2	23
3	21
4	17
5	11
6	5
7	2
8	1

2.3a What is the scale of measurement by which this variable was measured?

2.3b Is this variable (pits/quadrate) discrete or continuous?

2.3c Construct a bar graph of these data.

2.3d What is the total number of ant lion pits in all of the sampled quadrates?

2.4 Some species of chironomid larvae inhabit the leaves of pitcher plants. The number of larvae per leaf in a random sample of 197 leaves were as follows.

Larvae/Leaf (x)	Number of Leaves Containing x Number of Larvae
0	10
1	15
2	27
3	18
4	38
5	57
6	22
7	5
8	2
9	3
10	0

2.4a What is the scale of measurement by which this variable was measured?

2.4b Is this variable (larvae/leaf) continuous or discrete?

2.4c Construct a bar graph of these data.

2.4d What is the total number of chironomid larvae found in these 197 leaves?

2.5 Garter snakes respond to an overhead moving object by exhibiting an "escape" response. The intensity of this response may be measured on a somewhat subjective scale ranging from 3 to 0. A rapid movement of the snake from one location to another is given a score of 3, a movement involving at least one-third of the snake's body but not resulting in relocation of the animal is given a score of 2, a slight movement of the head only is given a score of 1, and no visible response is given a score of 0. Fifteen snakes were tested for this response and received the following scores:

3	2	3
1	3	2
3	3	1
0	2	3
2	0	2

2.5a What scale of measurement was used to obtain these data?

2.5b If you consider it appropriate to construct a graph to represent these data, do so. If you do not consider it appropriate, explain why.

2.6 Convert the following male heights (given in centimeters) into an ordinal scale.

Male Number	1	2	3	4	5	6
Height	181	202	190	185	190	200

2.7 Classify any male from exercise 2.6 who is less than 200 cm to be "short" and any male who is 200 cm or taller to be "tall," and convert the data into a nominal measurement.

2.8 Convert the following number of bullfrogs per pond into an ordinal scale.

Pond Number	1	2	3	4	5	6	7	8	9	10	11
Bullfrogs	34	65	23	34	18	20	15	70	15	18	34

2.9 Classify any pond that has 30 or fewer bullfrogs as "sparsely populated" and any pond that has more than 30 bullfrogs as "densely populated," and convert the data into a nominal scale.

2.10 For the following situations, identify the variable; indicate the scale of measurement; determine if the variable is discrete or continuous; and decide if the variable is simple, derived, or transformed.

2.10a The velocity of an enzyme-catalyzed reaction of substrate in micromoles converted per milligram of protein per minute.

2.10b The number of male bullfrogs in a pond and the number of female bullfrogs in the same pond (use caution in identifying the variable).

2.10c   The number of bullfrogs per hectare in several one-hectare quadrates.

2.10d   pH and pK_a.

2.10e   The velocity of snails, in furlongs per fortnight.

*2.11   Using the data on the lengths of bluegill sunfish in table B.1 (see appendix B), construct a histogram of the frequency distribution of this variable. A 10 mm class interval is recommended.

*2.12   Using the data on the length of female mosquito fish in table B.2, construct a histogram of the frequency distribution of this variable. A class interval of 4 mm is suggested.

*2.13   Using the data on pulse rate in table B.3, construct a histogram of the frequency distribution of this variable (for males and females).

*2.14   Using the data on pulse rate in table B.3, construct a histogram of the pulse rate of females.

*2.15   Using the data on pulse rate in table B.3, construct a histogram of the pulse rate of males.

Descriptive Statistics: Measures of Central Tendency and Dispersion

If we make measurements on a number of individuals in a population, we are very likely to find that not all individuals are alike with respect to the characteristic we are measuring. In fact we might find that no two are exactly alike with respect to this or any of a number of other measurable attributes. Among living organisms this variation from one individual to another is particularly noticeable. If we continue to examine our measurements, we may discover that there are certain values around which many, if not most, of our measurements tend to cluster. Statistics gives us ways to describe this tendency to cluster around some value (if such a tendency exists), and to describe the variation of individuals away from this central tendency. In this chapter we will consider several ways to describe the central tendency and the variation around it.

MEASURES OF CENTRAL TENDENCY

Several values may be used to describe the **central tendency** of a sample or a population. Which is most appropriate depends on the scale of measurement used and on the information we wish to convey.

The Mode

With data measured on a nominal scale, the only measure of central tendency is the **mode,** which is defined as the most frequent item in the data set. For example, in a group of 15 red marbles, 10 white marbles, and 5 blue marbles, the mode is red marbles.

The Median (M)

This is a useful measure of central tendency when data are measured on at least an ordinal scale. The items are arranged in order from smallest to largest. The **median** is the value that has an equal number of items above and below it. For example, in the measurements

$$2, 2, 2, 3, 3, 4, 4,$$

3 is the median, since this value has an equal number of measurements above and below it. When there are an even number of observations, none can have an equal number above and below. In this case the median is the value halfway between the two central values. In the series

$$2, 2, 2, 3, 4, 4, 4, 4,$$

the median is 3.5. Note that in the series

$$1, 2, 2, 3, 4, 10, 100, 1,000,$$

the median is still 3.5, even though the second series of numbers has a great deal more spread (dispersion) and covers a much larger range than the first.

The median is most often determined for ordinal data, but clearly one can also determine the median for data measured on an interval or ratio scale, and it is sometimes useful to do so.

The Arithmetic Mean (μ, $\bar{x}$)

The **arithmetic mean** is the most common measurement of central tendency when data are measured on an interval or ratio scale. It is sometimes also called the "mean" or "average." Note that in the above heading there are two symbols, μ and $\overline{x}$, used for the arithmetic mean. Why is this? If we measure all of the individuals in a population of interest and compute a mean based on these measurements, we have in fact obtained the true population mean; this is called the population or parametric mean, and it is symbolized by the Greek letter μ. On the other hand, if we measure only a randomly selected portion (sample) of the members of the population and use these measurements to compute a mean, we have obtained a sample mean, which is symbolized by $\overline{x}$.

If x_1, x_2, x_3, . . . , x_n are individual measurements, their mean (μ, $\overline{x}$) is

$$\mu = \frac{\Sigma x}{n} \quad \text{or} \quad \overline{x} = \frac{\Sigma x}{n} \tag{3.1}$$

or, in words, the sum of all of the x values divided by the total number of x values.

MEASURES OF DISPERSION

It is unlikely that individuals of a biological population will all be exactly alike in any variable that one cares to measure. We usually find that individuals differ from one another with respect to such things as length, weight, number of warts, and so on, but that there is some value about which individual measurements tend to cluster. When measuring with an interval or ratio scale, this value is the arithmetic mean, and when measuring with an ordinal scale this value is (sometimes) the median.

Consider the data in example 2.4 on length of male mosquito fish. The histogram of this frequency distribution is reproduced below as figure 3.1.

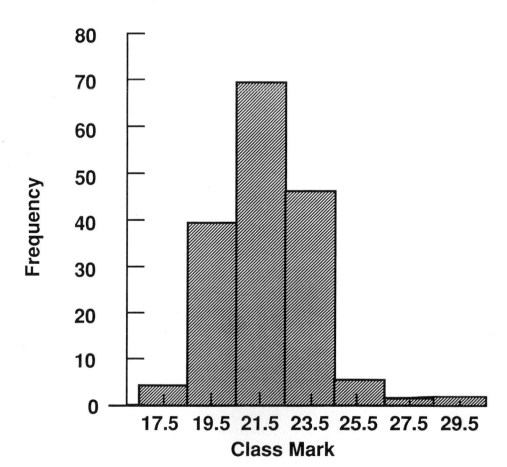

Figure 3.1
Frequency distribution of male
mosquito fish length (data from
example 2.4).

The mean for this sample is 21.84 mm. Note that the most frequently occurring size class is made up of individuals whose size clusters about the mean value. Note also that there are progressively fewer individuals in each size class as we move from the mean toward either smaller or larger individuals. Frequently, we have a need to measure this spread (or dispersion) of the individual observations around the mean.

The Range

This is a simple but not very useful measure of dispersion. The **range** is the difference between the largest and the smallest items in the sample. It is expressed in the same units as the original measurement. For example, the smallest measurement in the data on male mosquito fish length (table 2.3) is 17 mm, and the largest is 30 mm. The range is therefore 30 mm − 17 mm, or 13 mm. The range is strongly influenced by even a single extreme value, and it is therefore quite limited as an accurate description of the amount by which any individual measurement is likely to vary from the mean.

The Standard Deviation (σ, s)

The range as a measure of dispersion has the disadvantage that it takes into consideration only 2 items in the distribution—those 2 that differ from the mean by the greatest amount. A really useful measure of dispersion, and therefore of variation, must take into account all of the observations in a distribution. The **standard deviation** does exactly this. In effect it is a measure of the average amount by which each observation in a series of observations differs from the mean. We will use an imaginary set of data to illustrate the calculation and meaning of the standard deviation. We will assume that the measurements were made on an interval or ratio scale, since the following operations cannot be done with ordinal or nominal measurements. For now, assume that we are measuring all of these things that exist in the known universe. The measurements are these:

$$1, 2, 2, 3, 3, 4, 4, 5$$

The mean of these 8 measurements is

$$\mu = \frac{1 + 2 + 2 + 3 + 3 + 4 + 4 + 5}{8} = \frac{24}{8} = 3$$

We could compute an average deviation by first subtracting each observation (variant) from the mean, then summing these values and dividing by the number of observations. However, we would find that the sum of these values, symbolized by d, would equal zero (table 3.1), and the average deviation of the observations from the mean would therefore be zero. In fact, we would find that the sum of the deviates around any mean is always zero! Squaring each deviate eliminates the negative signs. When the squared deviates are summed, the resulting value is called the **sum of squares,** which we will abbreviate as SS.

The sum of squares may be obtained by squaring the difference between each observation and the mean of all of the observations, and then summing the squared differences, or

$$SS = \Sigma(x - \overline{x})^2 \tag{3.2}$$

As we shall see later, this is a very important quantity in many statistical procedures. In our example the sum of squares is 12 (see table 3.1). The procedure of subtracting each observation from the mean, squaring the difference, and summing these squared deviates is computationally very tedious if more than a few observations are involved. A much more efficient method of computing the sum of squares is:

$$SS = \Sigma x^2 - \frac{(\Sigma x)^2}{n} \qquad (3.3)$$

The first term in the equation, Σx^2, instructs one to square each observation and then sum the results. The second term, $\frac{(\Sigma x)^2}{n}$, instructs one to sum the observations, square the sum, and then divide the result by the number of observations.

If the sum of squares is divided by the number of observations, another important value, called the **variance,** is obtained:

$$\sigma^2 = variance = \frac{SS}{n} \qquad (3.4)$$

The variance represents the average of the squared deviations in a population or sample and therefore does not give us a very useful picture of the variation within the population or sample. To rectify this condition, we need only take the square root of the variance. This value is called the standard deviation, symbolized by the Greek letter σ.

$$\sigma = standard\ deviation = \sqrt{\frac{SS}{n}} = \sqrt{variance}. \qquad (3.5)$$

In our example the standard deviation is 1.225. Work through this example, which is summarized in table 3.1, to make certain that you thoroughly comprehend these concepts!

Table 3.1 Calculation of Mean, Variance, and Standard Deviation for a Population

x	d	d^2
1	-2	4
2	-1	1
2	-1	1
3	0	0
3	0	0
4	1	1
4	1	1
5	2	4
	$\Sigma = 0$	$SS = 12$

$$\sigma^2 = variance = 1.5$$
$$\sigma = standard\ deviation = 1.225$$

SAMPLE STATISTICS AND POPULATION PARAMETERS

It would be an unusual event indeed to have all of a population available for measurement. Even if we did, we might not want to take all the trouble to measure so many things. Thus, we generally do not know the true mean of a population, nor can we calculate the true variance. Accordingly, we calculate the mean and variance of a random sample from the population of interest and use them to estimate the population values. These values in the population as a whole are called **parameters,** and they are usually unknown. In a sample they are called **statistics** (plural; the singular is statistic). Thus, the true mean of a population is a parameter, and the mean of a sample taken from that population is a statistic. The sample statistic is an estimate of the population parameter. Parameters are conventionally symbolized by Greek letters and statistics by Roman letters, in this manner:

	parameter	*statistic*
mean	μ	$\bar{x}$
variance	σ^2	s^2
standard deviation	σ	s

The equations given above for computing variance and standard deviation are appropriate only when the entire population of interest has been measured. When the variance or standard deviation of samples are calculated as estimates of the true population values, it is more accurate to use equations 3.6 and 3.7:

$$s^2 = \frac{SS}{n - 1} \tag{3.6}$$

$$s = \sqrt{\frac{SS}{n - 1}} \tag{3.7}$$

Keep in mind that equations 3.4 and 3.5 are used for computing the population variance and standard deviation, and they can be used only when the entire population of interest is measured. In table 3.1 the population variance and standard deviation were calculated, since we assumed that our data included all of the members of a population. In table 3.2 the sample variance and standard deviation are given using equations 3.6 and 3.7.

Table 3.2   Calculation of Mean, Variance, and Standard Deviation for a Sample

x	d	d^2
1	-2	4
2	-1	1
2	-1	1
3	0	0
3	0	0
4	1	1
4	1	1
5	2	4
	$\Sigma = 0$	$SS = 12$

s^2 = variance = 1.7143

s = standard deviation = 1.3093

Why we use n as the denominator in equations 3.4 and 3.5 and $n - 1$ in equations 3.6 and 3.7 might be confusing. This is based on the concept of statistical independence. Keep in mind that equations 3.4 and 3.5 measure parameters, while equations 3.6 and 3.7 are estimates of these parameters. Statisticians tell us that dividing by $n - 1$, called **degrees of freedom,** gives a more accurate (unbiased) estimate.

COMPUTER SUPPLEMENT

Virtually all statistical programs for computers give summary statistics for a sample variable. The summary statistics for the length of male mosquito fish from example 2.4 (see chapter 2), as computed by MINITAB, are shown in figure 3.2. In this printout, "TRMEAN" is the "trimmed mean," which is the

```
:MTB > describe c1
:            N      MEAN    MEDIAN    TRMEAN     STDEV    SEMEAN
:C1         172    21.901    22.000    21.799     2.065     0.157
:
:            MIN      MAX        Q1        Q3
:C1       17.000   31.000    20.000    23.000
:MTB >
```

Figure 3.2
MINITAB printout of the summary statistics for example 2.4.

mean computed after the smallest 5% and the largest 5% of the observations have been removed. "Q1" and "Q3" are the first and third quartiles, which, together with the median, effectively divide the observations into four groups, each containing one-fourth of the observations.

KEY TERMS

arithmetic mean
central tendency
degrees of freedom
median
mode
parameter

range
standard deviation
statistics
sum of squares
variance

EXERCISES

(Exercises preceded by an asterisk are suitable for a computer solution.)

3.1 For the following sample, compute the mean, median, range, sum of squares, variance, and standard deviation.

$$2 \quad 5 \quad 3 \quad 7 \quad 8 \quad 3 \quad 9 \quad 3 \quad 10 \quad 4 \quad 7 \quad 4 \quad 6 \quad 11 \quad 9$$
$$9 \quad 11 \quad 5 \quad 7 \quad 3 \quad 8 \quad 9 \quad 2 \quad 1 \quad 3 \quad 8 \quad 3 \quad 8 \quad 9 \quad 3$$

3.2 For the following sample, compute the mean, median, range, sum of squares, variance, and standard deviation.

$$23 \quad 43 \quad 12 \quad 56 \quad 43 \quad 23 \quad 56 \quad 43 \quad 23 \quad 32 \quad 12 \quad 14 \quad 15$$

3.3 For the following sample, compute the mean, median, range, sum of squares, and standard deviation.

$$23 \quad 76 \quad 98 \quad 78 \quad 65 \quad 23 \quad 43 \quad 54 \quad 37 \quad 65 \quad 47 \quad 80 \quad 92 \quad 35$$
$$9 \quad 78 \quad 67 \quad 65 \quad 56 \quad 43 \quad 12 \quad 87 \quad 67 \quad 35 \quad 63 \quad 12 \quad 89 \quad 12$$

3.4 A random sample of 42 belted kingfishers was collected from various locations in North America and their culmen (bill) lengths were measured in millimeters. The data are these:

48.1	50.8	48.8	56.8	57.7	47.0
56.8	60.2	55.8	59.2	52.5	50.4
48.0	57.1	51.8	52.3	47.8	58.0
53.4	55.2	51.0	59.3	61.5	61.2
57.8	50.1	56.0	56.5	55.8	56.5
56.3	59.8	61.8	56.2	57.5	59.3
62.4	61.1	59.9	55.6	56.8	59.2

Compute the mean, median, range, sum of squares, variance, and standard deviation for this sample.

3.5 Using the data from exercise 2.1 (see chapter 2), compute the mean, sum of squares, variance, and standard deviation for the sample of 148 male heights.

3.6 Using the data from exercise 2.2, compute the mean, sum of squares, variance, and standard deviation for this sample of largemouth bass lengths.

3.7 Using samples of 10, 20, and 30 bluegill sunfish standard lengths from exercise 1.1 (see chapter 1), compute the mean and standard deviation of each. Consider the measurements in table B.1 (see appendix B) to be the entire population of interest, with a population mean of 120.03 mm and a population standard deviation of 41.95 mm. Are the sample means and standard deviations of your samples the same as the population mean and standard deviation? Why do you suppose that there might be a difference in the sample values and the population values? Save your calculated values for later use.

3.8 Using the samples of 10, 20, and 30 male mosquito fish lengths from exercise 1.3, compute the sample mean and standard deviation of each sample. Consider the measurements in table B.2 to be the entire population of interest, with a population mean of 23.60 mm and a population standard deviation of 2.64 mm. Are the sample means and standard deviations the same as the population mean and standard deviation? How do you account for the difference? Save your calculated values for later use.

3.9 Using the samples of 10, 20, and 30 female mosquito fish lengths from exercise 1.3, compute the mean, sum of squares, variance, and standard deviation for these samples. Consider the measurements in table B.2 to be the entire population of interest, with a population mean of 34.29 mm and a population standard deviation of 5.49 mm. Are the means and standard deviations of your samples the same as the population mean and standard deviation? How do you account for the difference? Save your calculated values for later use.

3.10 Using the samples of 10, 20, and 30 pulse rates from exercise 1.4, compute the mean and standard deviation of each. Consider the measurements in table B.3 to be the entire population of interest, with a population mean of 78.81 and a population standard deviation of 13.51. Are the sample means and standard deviations of your samples the same as the population mean and standard deviation? Why do you suppose there might be a difference in the sample values and the population values? Save your calculated values for later use.

3.11 Using the samples of 10, 20, and 30 reaction times from exercise 1.5, compute the mean and standard deviation of each. Consider the measurements in table B.3 to be the entire population of interest, with a population mean of 179.67 msec and a population standard deviation of 40.43 msec. Are the sample means and standard deviations of your samples the same as the population mean and standard deviation? Why do you suppose that there might be a difference in the sample values and the population values? Save your calculated values for later use.

3.12 Using the data from exercise 2.5, select and compute an appropriate measure of central tendency.

3.13 Using the data from exercise 2.3, compute the mean number of ant lion pits/quadrate for this sample. Save your calculated value for later use.

3.14 Using the data from exercise 2.4, compute the mean number of chironomid larvae per pitcher plant leaf. Save your calculated value for later use.

For exercises 3.15 through 3.19, consider the data in tables B.1 through B.3 to be large samples.

*3.15 Using the data from table B.1, compute the mean, variance, and standard deviation of bluegill sunfish length.

*3.16 Using the data from table B.2, compute the mean, variance, and standard deviation of total lengths of male mosquito fish.

*3.17 Using the data from table B.2, compute the mean, variance, and standard deviation of total lengths of female mosquito fish.

*3.18 Using the data from table B.3, compute the mean, variance, and standard deviation of human pulse rates.

*3.19 Using the data from table B.3, compute the mean, variance, and standard deviation of human reaction times.

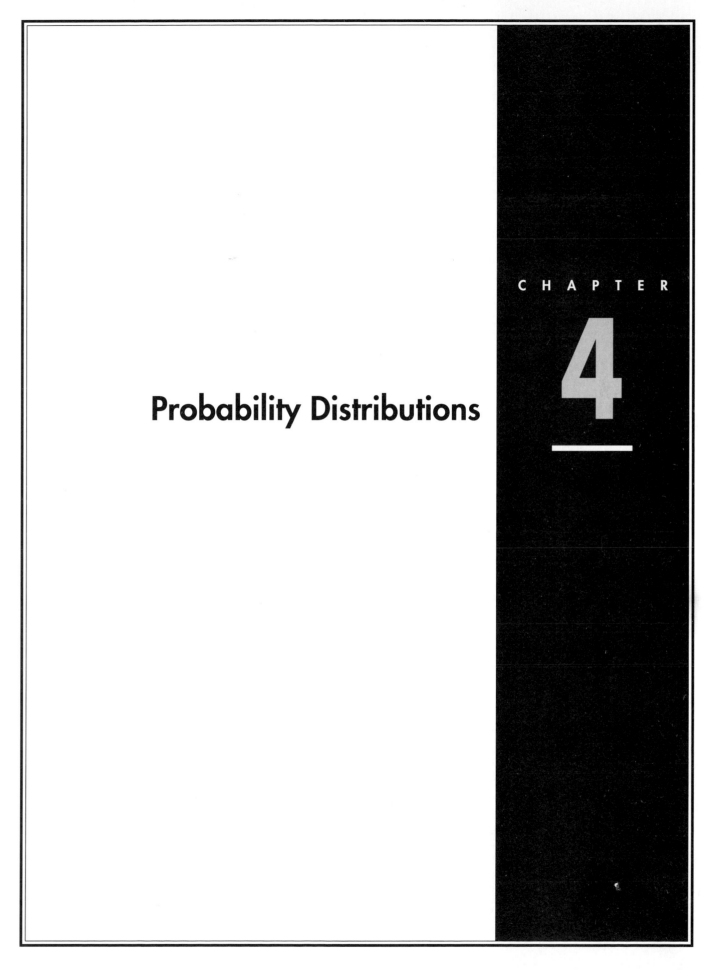

Probability Distributions

In this chapter we will consider some of the basic rules of probability and some important probability distributions. Although we will not deal with probability in a formal way, several of the basic rules of probability are introduced in this chapter as they are needed.

The probability of some event is the chance or likelihood that that event will occur, expressed numerically as between zero and one (or, in common usage, as between zero and 100%). A probability near one suggests that the event is very likely, while a probability near zero suggests that the event is very unlikely. Note that once an event has occurred, there is no longer a probability associated with it. The probability that lightning might strike a particular tree on any given day might be very small, but once the tree has been struck on that particular day, thinking of the probability of this happening is meaningless!

There are several ways of arriving at the probability of an event, but only two of these need concern us here. One way is empirical and is based on some prior knowledge of the event in the population of interest. For example, if we know that 3 out of every 5 individuals in a population is a female, then we may state that the probability that any individual selected at random from this population will be a female is $\frac{3}{5}$, or 0.6. Note that in this case, we required knowledge of the specific population of interest to arrive at this probability.

A second important way of arriving at a probability for an event is based on a theoretical consideration. Dice have 6 faces, each bearing a number of 1 through 6. Given that a die is "fair" (that is, equally as likely to land with one face up as any other), then the probability of obtaining any particular number on the toss of a single die is $\frac{1}{6}$ or 0.1667. We need toss no dice to arrive at this probability.

Note that in both of these cases, the probability was calculated from a ratio. This is the first of our probability rules, called the division rule.

The Division Rule

The probability of an event is the number of ways that an event can occur divided by the total number of events that may occur.

In the first case, there were 3 ways that a female could occur out of every 5 possible occurrences of an individual of either sex. In the second case, there was one way that a particular number could occur out of 6 possible occurrences.

A **probability distribution** is exactly what the name indicates: a distribution of probabilities. In chapter 2 we encountered frequency distributions of different kinds of variables. These were constructed from actual measurements of how often (the frequency) a certain event occurred (how often a male mosquito fish with a length between 18.5 mm and 20.5 mm occurred, how often a quadrate containing 2 maple seedlings occurred, and so on).

Probability distributions are exactly the same thing, except that they plot the *probability* of a certain event rather than the actual occurrence (frequency) of that event. Thus, they are not based on actual occurrences but on calculated probabilities that these events will occur given that certain assumptions are true. If we toss a coin, there are 2 possible outcomes—a head or a tail. On any given toss, there is an equal chance of obtaining a head or a tail because the coin has an equal number of heads and tails—one of each—

and because the 2 possible outcomes are mutually exclusive. The outcome can be only one or the other. Thus, the probability that any toss of the coin will produce a head is 1 (the outcome of interest) divided by 2 (the number of possible outcomes), or $\frac{1}{2}$ (or 0.5). The probability that any toss will result in a tail is, of course, also $\frac{1}{2}$ (or 0.5) and is deduced in the same manner as above. Or we may compute the probability of a tail in this manner: let $p =$ the probability of a head and $q =$ the probability of a tail. Since the probability that the outcome will be one or the other (a head or a tail) is $\frac{2}{2} = 1.00$, then

$$p + q = 1, \text{ and}$$
$$q = 1 - p, \text{ or}$$
$$q = 1 - 0.5 = 0.5$$

A probability distribution that describes this situation is:

Outcome	Probability
head	0.5
tail	0.5

A graph of this probability distribution is shown in figure 4.1.

Note that we need toss no coins to arrive at this probability distribution. It is a theoretical distribution that we derive from our knowledge of how

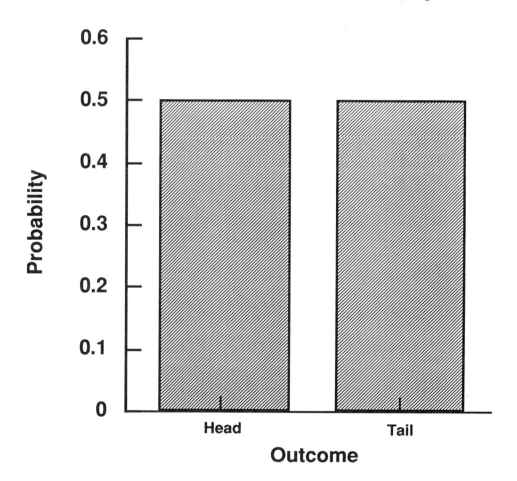

Figure 4.1
Probability distribution of the outcomes of the toss of a single coin.

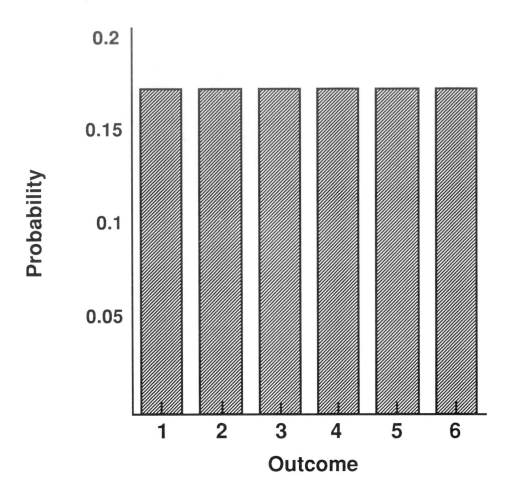

Figure 4.2
Probability distribution of the outcomes of the toss of a single die.

flipped coins behave and from the laws of probability. Such a probability distribution is useful in many ways, not the least of which is to predict what we expect to happen in the real world. If we tossed a coin 100 times, we would expect to obtain approximately 50 heads and 50 tails if our assumptions about coin behavior under these conditions are correct. If we toss a die, the probability of obtaining a 1 is $\frac{1}{6}$ (0.1666), the probability of obtaining a 2 is $\frac{1}{6}$ (0.1666), and so on, for each of the 6 possible outcomes. The probability distribution for the outcomes of a toss of a die is shown in figure 4.2.

Again, note that we do not have to roll a lot of dice to arrive at this probability distribution. We deduce it from our knowledge of dice and the laws of probability. It is not based on observations of real events.

DISCRETE PROBABILITY DISTRIBUTIONS

Several probability distributions describe the behavior of discrete variables. Two of these—the binomial distribution and the Poisson distribution—are considered in this chapter.

The Binomial Distribution

Many objects or events might be thought of as belonging to one of two mutually exclusive categories. Heads or tails, male or female, present or absent, sick or well, and asleep or awake are obvious examples. Even when there are more than two mutually exclusive categories, it is sometimes possible and useful to "lump" various categories into two by considering the object or event of interest as one category and everything else as the other category. Thus, "red" and "not red" are two mutually exclusive categories, even though "not red" can consist of blue, green, yellow, or any of a large number of colors that are not red. In the toss of a die, we might designate "1" as one possible outcome and "not 1" (any result except 1) as the other alternative.

The **binomial probability distribution** describes the probabilities associated with the outcome of certain events that have the following properties. You will need to refer back to these properties from time to time, since they are likely to be a bit confusing until you gain some experience and insight by way of the examples and problems that follow.

Properties of the Binomial Probability Distribution

1. The event (the toss of a coin, for example), sometimes called a trial, occurs a specified number of times, designated as k.
2. Each time the event occurs, there are 2 mutually exclusive outcomes (a head or a tail). One of these outcomes is specified as the outcome of interest (sometimes arbitrarily called a "success"). The probability of this outcome is designated as p. The probability of the other outcome (a "failure" in statistical jargon) is designated as q. Since there are only 2 possible outcomes, $p + q = 1$ and $q = 1 - p$.
3. The events (trials) are independent, meaning that the outcome of one event has no influence on the outcome of other events in the series of events.
4. The number of times that the outcome of interest (a "success") occurs in k events (trials) is designated as x. The binomial probability distribution gives the probabilities of x, symbolized by $p(x)$, for values of x from zero to k.

Consider the possible events that can take place when you toss 2 coins simultaneously. The result can be 2 heads, 1 head and 1 tail, or 2 tails. What would the probability distribution for this situation look like? In other words, what is the probability of each of the 3 possible outcomes? The probability that one coin will be a head is 0.5 ($\frac{1}{2}$), and the probability that the other coin will be a head is also 0.5 (note that these 2 probabilities are independent of each other—the way that one coin lands has no effect on the way that the other coin lands). The probability that both will be heads is the product of their individual probabilities, which is 0.5 $\times$ 0.5, or 0.25.

The Multiplication Rule (the "And" Rule)

The probability that independent events will occur simultaneously (that event A *and* event B will both occur) is the product of the probabilities that the events will occur individually. Stated another way: if A and B are independent events with probabilities $p(A)$ and $p(B)$, the probability of the joint occurrence of both A and B is $p(A \text{ and } B) = p(A)p(B)$.

In the same manner, we determine the probability of 2 tails to be 0.25. However, there are 2 ways that the occurrence of one head and one tail can result. The first coin can be a tail ($p = 0.5$) and the second coin can be a head ($p = 0.5$), and the probability of this result is 0.5 $\times$ 0.5, or 0.25; on the other hand, the first coin can be a head ($p = 0.5$) and the second coin can be a tail ($p = 0.5$). The probability of this result is, as before, 0.25. Now since the probability of a head and a tail is 0.25 and the probability of a tail and a head is 0.25, the probability of this event happening in either one of these 2 ways is $0.25 + 0.25 = 0.5$.

The Addition Rule (the "Or" Rule)

The probability that at least one of 2 or more alternative outcomes will occur is the sum of the individual probabilities that the events will occur. In other words, if A and B are independent events with probabilities p(A) and p(B), the probability that either event A or event B will occur is p(A or B) = p(A) + p(B).

It might help to visualize this situation graphically, as shown below. The rows represent the possible outcomes of one coin, and the columns represent the possible outcomes of the other coin. We compute the probabilities of the possible joint occurrences of the 2 coins simply by multiplying the columns by the rows. (This approach may remind you of the Punnett square treatment in genetics. That is because it is the same concept!)

		The Other Coin	
		H ($p = 0.5$)	T ($p = 0.5$)
	H ($p = 0.5$)	HH	HT
One Coin		($p = 0.5 \times 0.5$)	($p = 0.5 \times 0.5$)
	T ($p = 0.5$)	TH	TT
		($p = 0.5 \times 0.5$)	($p = 0.5 \times 0.5$)

A bar graph of the probability distribution for this situation is shown in figure 4.3.

We may deduce these probabilities in an intuitive manner, as we did above, or we may simply expand the binomial expression:

$$(p + q)^k = 1 \tag{4.1}$$

in which p is the probability of one outcome of interest (heads), q is the probability of the other outcome (tails), and k is the number of events (trials or occurrences). In our example, p is 0.5 (the probability that any coin toss will result in a head), q is $1 - p$ ($1 - 0.5 = 0.5$), and k is 2 (the number of coins tossed). Expanding the binomial expression above gives

$$p^2 + 2pq + q^2 = 1, \text{ or } 0.25 + 0.50 + 0.25$$

Each term in the expanded binomial expression gives the probability of one of the possible outcomes. Note that these probabilities are the same as those we deduced earlier with a more intuitive approach.

What are the probabilities of the various outcomes when 3 coins are tossed ($k = 3$)? The possible outcomes are: 3 heads, 2 heads and 1 tail, 1 head and 2 tails, and 3 tails. As before, p (the probability that any coin will be a head) is 0.5, and q is $1 - p$, or 0.5. Expanding the binomial expression

$$(p + q)^3 = 1 \text{ gives}$$

$$p^3 + 3p^2q + 3pq^2 + q^3 = 1, \text{ or}$$

$$0.125 + 0.375 + 0.375 + 0.125 = 1$$

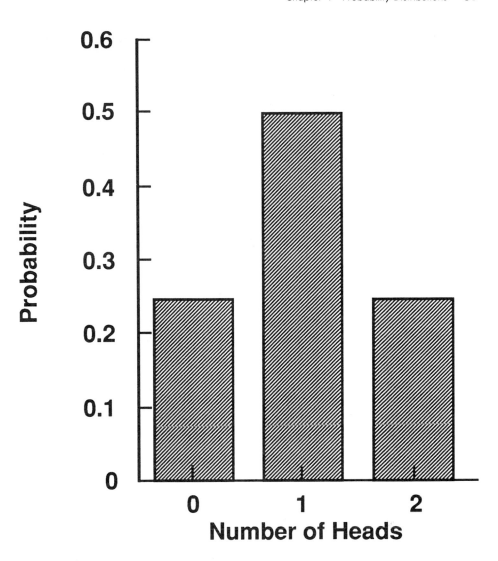

Figure 4.3
Binomial probability
distribution for k = 2 *and*
p = 0.5.

These then are the probabilities associated with each of the 4 possible outcomes (0.125 for 3 heads, 0.375 for 2 heads and 1 tail, and so on). This probability distribution is shown as a bar graph in figure 4.4.

You may recall from high school algebra that expanding binomial expressions is not a lot of fun, especially when k becomes large. Fortunately there is a better way. The probability of the occurrence of x events of interest (heads, for example), symbolized by $p(x)$, in k trials (coins tossed, for example), is given by equation 4.2.

$$p(x) = \frac{k!}{x!(k-x)!} p^x q^{(k-x)} \qquad (4.2)$$

where k is the number of trials (coins tossed), x is the number of occurrences of the event of interest whose probability we wish to predict (the number of heads), and p is the probability associated with the occurrence of x (0.5 in this case). How is equation 4.2 used? Some examples will help to illustrate this.

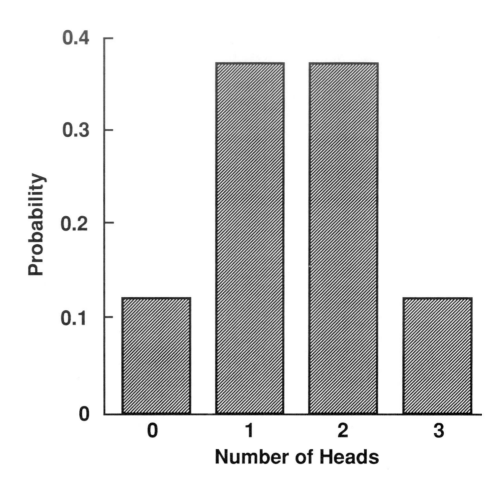

Figure 4.4
Binomial probability
distribution for k = 3 *and*
p = 0.5.

EXAMPLE 4.1   Calculating a Binomial Probability

Suppose we wish to know the probability of obtaining 1 head in the toss of 3 coins (either 3 coins tossed simultaneously or 1 coin tossed 3 times in succession—in other words, in 3 trials). In this case $x = 1$ (the number of heads in which we have an interest), $k = 3$ (the number of trials), $p = 0.5$ (the probability associated with event x), and $q = 1 - p = 0.5$.   ∎

Substituting these values in equation 4.2 gives:

$$p(x) = \frac{3!}{1!(3 - 1)!} \, 0.5^1 \times 0.5^2 = 0.375$$

To verify that you understand the use of equation 4.2, find $p(x)$ for the other 3 possible outcomes in this situation (the probability of 0 heads and 3 tails is 0.125, of 1 head and 2 tails is 0.375, of 2 heads and 1 tail is 0.375, and of 3 heads and 0 tails is 0.125). Remember that by definition **0! = 1.**

So far we have considered only situations in which p and q are equal (both 0.5). This is not always the case. Consider the probability distribution of obtaining x number of ones in the toss of 2 dice. We will consider a "1" to be one event of interest and "not 1" as the other event. The probability of obtaining any particular number on the roll of a single die is $\frac{1}{6}$ (0.1667); thus, p (the probability of a 1) is 0.1667, and q (the probability of obtaining any

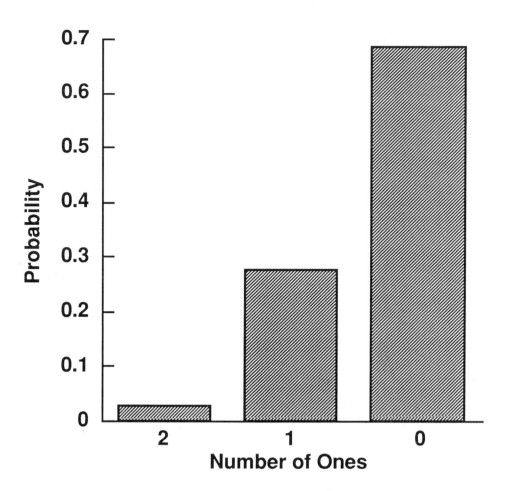

Figure 4.5
Binomial probability
distribution for k = 2 *and*
p = 0.1667.

result except 1) is $1 - 0.1667$, or 0.8333. Since we are tossing 2 dice in this experiment, $k = 2$. Substituting these values in equations 4.1 or 4.2 gives these results:

Number of "Ones" (x)	Number of "Not Ones"	p(x)
2	0	.03
1	1	.28
0	2	.69

Thus, the probability of obtaining 2 ones in a toss of 2 dice is only 0.03 (or approximately 3 times in 100 tosses). This probability distribution is shown as a bar graph in figure 4.5. Compare this with figure 4.1, the probability distribution for $k = 2$ and both p and $q = 0.5$.

Of what practical use is the binomial distribution to us as biologists? Perhaps some examples will serve to illustrate some of the many ways we use this particular probability distribution.

EXAMPLE 4.2   A Binomial Variable

Bush hogs always have litters of 6 hoglets. We will assume, based on our theoretical knowledge of the genetics of sex determination, that the probability that any hoglet in a litter will be a male is 0.5 and the probability that any hoglet will be a female is also 0.5. We wish to know how many litters in 100 litters will consist of 5 or more males, if our assumption about the equal probability of an individual hoglet being a male or a female is correct. ∎

Note that this problem is exactly equivalent to asking how often we would obtain 5 or more heads in the toss of 6 coins. First we solve equation 4.2 for $x = 5$, which is:

$$p(5) = \frac{6!}{5! \times 1!} \, 0.5^5 \times 0.5^1 = 0.0939$$

Thus, the probability associated with exactly 5 males in a litter of 6 is 0.0939. However, our question asked for the probability associated with 5 *or more* males in a litter of 6. So we must also determine the probability associated with 6 males in a litter, which is:

$$p(6) = \frac{6!}{6! \times 0!} \, 0.5^6 \times 0.5^0 = 0.0156$$

The probability associated with exactly 6 males in a litter of 6 is 0.0156. The probability associated with either 5 *or* 6 males in a litter of 6 is $p(5) +$ $p(6)$, which is

$$0.0939 + 0.0156 = 0.1095$$

In 100 litters we would therefore expect to find 100×0.1095—approximately 11 litters—consisting of 5 or more male hoglets.

EXAMPLE 4.3 Example 4.2 Viewed in a Different Context

Let us ask the same question in a slightly different way: In 100 litters, how many consisting of each of the possible combinations of males and females would we expect to find (how many with 6 males and no females, with 5 males and 1 female, with 4 males and 2 females, and so on)? ■

For this solution we would simply solve equation 4.2 for each value of x from 6 to 0, and we would obtain the results shown in table 4.1.

Table 4.1 The Data for Example 4.3

Number of Males (x)	Number of Females (k − x)	p(x)	Expected Frequency p(x) × 100
6	0	0.0156	1.56
5	1	0.0938	9.38
4	2	0.2344	23.44
3	3	0.3125	31.25
2	4	0.2344	23.44
1	5	0.0938	9.38
0	6	0.0156	1.56

What use might we wish to make of such a probability distribution, which is based on theoretical assumptions rather than on real world observations? Consider example 4.2. Suppose we suspect that the gender of bush hoglets is not a matter of random chance but rather that some females tend to produce an inordinately large number of offspring of one sex or the other (a phenomenon that has actually been observed in a number of species). Suppose also that we actually surveyed 100 litters of bush hogs, each consisting of 6 hoglets, and found that 20 or so contained 5 or 6 male hoglets and a similar number contained 5 or 6 female hoglets. This is about twice as many as our binomial probability distribution predicts, and therefore, we would have reason to suspect that sex determination in this species is not a random event. In other words, some factor or factors other than the chance combination of X and Y chromosomes is involved.

Note carefully that without the prediction based on the binomial probability distribution, we would not know if the number of predominately one-sex litters that we observed was too large to be produced by random combinations of X and Y chromosomes. In other words, we cannot conclude that a result is not due to chance alone unless we know what result is expected if it is. This concept is the basis for much of statistical hypothesis testing, which is the subject of chapter 5.

The Poisson Distribution

Another discrete probability distribution often useful to biologists is the **Poisson distribution.** Generally we use the Poisson distribution to predict the probabilities of the occurrences of "rare" events (when such occurrences are known to be independent of one another) or to determine if the occurrences of such events are independent of one another. The event of interest must be rare, which is to say that its occurrence in any sampling unit must be small *relative to the number of times that it could occur,* and occurrences of the event must be independent of previous occurrences of the event in the sampling unit.

EXAMPLE 4.4   A Poisson Variable

In the maple seedling example in chapter 2 (reproduced below as table 4.2), most of the quadrates sampled had no seedlings, several had 1, a few had 2, and so on. We would like to know if the occurrences of maple seedlings are independent events. If so, their frequency of occurrence in the quadrates should follow a Poisson distribution. If they do not follow a Poisson distribution, we conclude that the events are not independent and that the occurrence of a maple seedling in a quadrate in some way influences the occurrences of other maple seedlings in that quadrate. ■

Table 4.2 Maple Seedlings per Quadrate

Number of Plants/Quadrate	Frequency
0	35
1	28
2	15
3	10
4	7
5	5

Since the number of seedlings that could conceivably occur in a quadrate is quite large, we may consider the observed frequencies to be rare events. If the presence of a seedling in a quadrate does not alter the possible occurrence of other seedlings in a quadrate, the frequency of seedlings per quadrate should follow a Poisson distribution. If there is a major deviation of the observed frequency distribution from the Poisson distribution, then we have reason to suspect that the occurrences of maple seedlings are not independent events, which is to say that the distribution of maple seedlings is not random, and that some factor or factors in the environment other than chance influences the distribution.

What the Poisson distribution predicts is how many units (quadrates, in this case) are expected to have no occurrences of the event (maple seedlings), how many are expected to have 1, how many are expected to have 2, and so on, if the events are rare and independent. These probabilities are given by the expression:

$$p(x) = \frac{\mu^x e^{-\mu}}{x!}$$

where μ is the population mean occurrence of the event per sampling unit, e is the base of natural logarithms (2.7183), and $p(x)$ is the probability of x events in a unit. Since we usually have no knowledge of the population mean, it is estimated by the sample mean, and $p(x)$ is computed by equation 4.3.

$$p(x) = \frac{\bar{x}^x e^{-\bar{x}}}{x!} \tag{4.3}$$

for probabilities, $p(x)$, of 0, 1, 2, 3, 4, and so on, occurrences per unit. In the maple seedling example, there were 100 quadrates (units) and a total of 141 seedlings (events) in these 100 quadrates. The mean number of occurrences ($\bar{x}$) was therefore $\frac{141}{100}$ or 1.41 plants per quadrate. Solving equation 4.3 for relative expected occurrences per unit (seedlings per quadrate) of 0, 1, 2, 3, 4, 5, and 6, gives the results shown in table 4.3 under the column designated "$p(x)$." Multiplying these values by the number of sampled units (100 in this case) gives the expected frequencies. The last column in the table gives the values that were actually observed. The column headed "Cumulative" is the cumulative probability for the designated value of x or any smaller value. It is occasionally convenient to make use of this cumulative distribution.

Table 4.3 Expected and Observed Frequencies of Maple Seedlings per Quadrate ($\bar{x} = 1.41$, n = 100)

Number/Quadrate (x)	p(x)	Cumulative	Expected	Observed
0	.244	.244	24.4	35
1	.344	.588	34.4	28
2	.243	.831	24.3	15
3	.114	.945	11.4	10
4	.040	.985	4.0	7
5	.011	.996	1.1	5

Figure 4.6 is a graphic representation of the expected distribution and the actual observed distribution from table 4.3. The expected distribution (i.e., the Poisson probability distribution) is the distribution we would expect if the maple seedlings were distributed randomly within the sampled habitat.

A frequent use of the Poisson distribution is in testing whether events are "clumped" or "repulsed" with respect to each other in space or time, or whether the events are occurring independently of one another and are therefore distributed randomly. Note in figure 4.6 that the expected (Poisson) distribution and the actual observed distribution do not match very well. We might suspect, therefore, that the occurrences of maple seedlings are not independent of one another. In chapter 9 we will discuss ways of determining if this difference is real or if it is simply the result of chance. Example 4.4 illustrates one way in which the Poisson distribution is commonly used in ecology. This distribution also finds use in many other situations. Example 4.5 illustrates how the Poisson distribution might be applied to a microbial genetics problem.

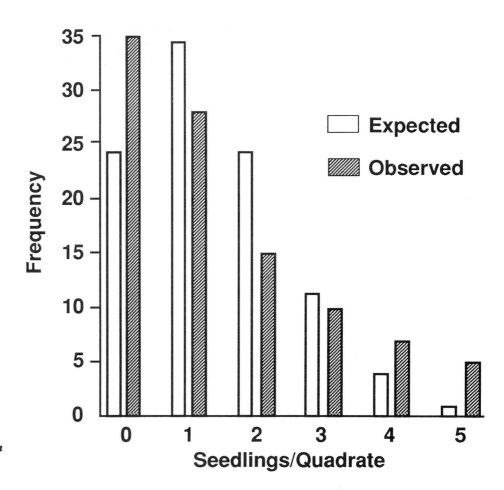

Figure 4.6
Poisson probability distribution
for $\bar{x}$ = 1.41.

EXAMPLE 4.5 A Poisson Variable

Bacterial viruses infect bacterial cells by first adsorbing onto the bacterial cell wall. The number of phage particles that adsorb to any one bacterial cell is a Poisson process. In a certain experiment, 2.5×10^6 phage particles were mixed with 10^6 bacterial cells. Thus, the mean number of phage particles per bacterial cell is 2.5. We wish to know what proportion of the bacterial culture would be expected to have no phage particles adsorbed to them. ∎

The mean number of phage particles per bacterial cell is 2.5. Substituting this value in equation 4.3 and solving for $p(0)$ gives:

$$p(0) = \frac{2.5^0 \times e^{-2.5}}{0!} = 0.0821$$

Thus, the probability that any randomly selected cell would have no phage particles adsorbed to it is 0.0821. This is also the proportion of the cells in the bacterial culture that would be expected to be free of phage particles. Obviously, then, the actual number of bacterial cells with no phage particles is expected to be $0.0821 \times 10^6 = 8.21 \times 10^4$.

A question like this can be asked in a different way. Suppose we wish to add a sufficient number of phage particles to a bacterial culture to ensure that not more than 1% (0.01) of the bacterial cells remain uninfected. How many phage particles would we need to add, assuming that we know or may determine the number of bacterial cells present? Could you suggest how this might be calculated? Exercises 4.34 and 4.35 at the end of this chapter are questions of this type.

THE NORMAL DISTRIBUTION

The **normal distribution** is one of several continuous probability distributions. Not only does it describe, in an approximate way, a large number of variables, but it also provides the conceptual basis of many statistical procedures.

Continuous variables can assume any value between certain limits. If drawn as a continuous line rather than as bars representing class intervals, the frequency distribution histogram of a continuous variable very often forms a symmetrical bell-shaped curve or something closely approximating such a curve. In theory, if we plotted the histogram using a very large (infinite) number of measurements and the smallest imaginable class interval, the histogram would become a smooth curve, somewhat like figure 4.7. If it helps, think of the curve as a frequency polygon of an infinitely large population with the smallest imaginable class interval. The probability distribution that describes distributions of this general type is the normal probability distribution, one of the most important theoretical distributions in statistics.

Some Properties of a Normal Distribution

The normal probability distribution is a theoretical mathematical concept whose derivation is well beyond our present concern or needs. However, we know that a large number of continuous variables encountered in nature tend to follow such a distribution. Many discrete variables also approximately follow such a distribution when the range of values that the variable may assume is fairly large (see ''Normal Approximation of the Binomial Distribution'' later in this chapter). The normal probability distribution has certain important characteristics, which are discussed below. Frequent reference to figure 4.8 will assist in understanding these characteristics.

Properties of the Normal Distribution

1. The distribution is completely defined by the mean (μ) and the standard deviation (σ). The location of the curve along the x-axis is defined by the mean, and the spread of the curve is defined by the standard deviation. Since these parameters can assume, theoretically, an infinity of values, there are an infinite number of normal distributions.
2. The height on the y-axis of any point along the curve represents the probability density function, $f(x)$, of that value of the variable. The probability density function is expressed formally as:

$$f(x) = \frac{1}{\sigma\sqrt{2\pi}} e^{1/2(x - \mu/\sigma)^2}$$

We cannot think of this y-axis value as representing a probability (or frequency) since a point has no dimension, and therefore, a line drawn vertically from such a point has no width. Thus, there is no real value that corresponds to this value of x. However, if we consider two values of x that are *very* close together, we may now

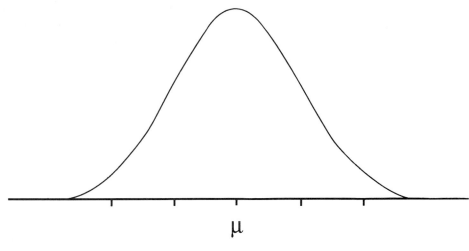

Figure 4.7
A normal distribution.

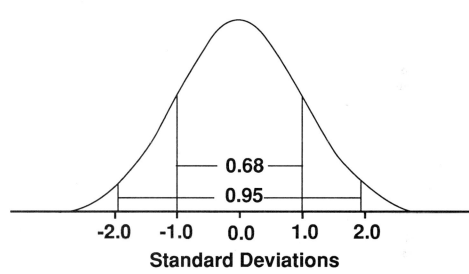

Figure 4.8
Areas of a normal distribution.

compute the area of the curve that lies between these two values. In this way we may assign a probability to a very narrow *range* (class interval) of the variable in question.

3. The curve is perfectly symmetrical about the mean. Thus, the mean and median are equal.

4. One standard deviation above the mean includes 34.13% of all of the individuals in the population, and one standard deviation below the mean includes 34.13% of all of the individuals in the population. Thus, 68.26% of all of the individuals in the population fall within plus or minus one standard deviation of the mean. Another way of thinking about this is that there is a probability of 0.6826 that any individual (x) taken at random from this population would fall within one standard deviation of the mean. In a similar manner, the mean ± 2 standard deviations contains 95.46% of all of the individuals in the population (or, the probability that any individual taken at random from this population would fall within ± 2 standard deviations of the mean is 0.9546). The mean ± 3 standard deviations contains 99.73% of all the individuals within the population (table 4.4 and figure 4.8). We will have occasion to examine this property in considerably more detail in this and subsequent chapters.

Table 4.4 Percentages of the Area of the Normal Curve as a Function of the Standard Deviation

Standard Deviations	Percent of Area
±1	68.26 (.6826)
±1.960	95 (.950)
±2	95.46 (.9546)
±2.576	99 (.99)
±3	99.73 (.9973)

The area under the normal curve is, by definition, 1. Since the normal curve is defined by the mean and the standard deviation, there is a fixed relationship between the standard deviation and the proportion of the area under the curve that occurs between the mean and any standard deviation "unit." The relationships shown in table 4.4 and figure 4.8 hold true for any normal distribution.

The Standard Normal Distribution

Fortunately, we do not have to deal with complex computations with the normal probability density function every time we wish to do something with the normal distribution. Among the infinite variety of normal distributions that are possible, there is one to which all others may be rather easily converted: the **standard normal distribution.** It has a mean of zero, a standard deviation and variance of one, and its "tails" extend from minus infinity (wherever that might be) through zero (the mean) to positive infinity. Table A.1 gives the proportion of the standard normal curve that lies between zero (the mean) and almost any value of a variable that one might reasonably expect to encounter. How this table is used is discussed in the examples that follow.

Some Uses of the Normal Distribution

The normal distribution has many applications in statistics. In the following example, we will explore only a few of the uses of this probability distribution. Others will become apparent in subsequent chapters.

We often need to determine where, on a normal curve, a particular value falls, or more often, the probability that some value or range of values lies within a certain portion of the curve. To do this, individual variants need to be expressed as if they were variants of the standard normal distribution. In other words, we need to convert our normal distribution, which may have any imaginable mean, variance, and standard deviation, to the standard normal distribution, which has a mean of zero and a variance and standard deviation of one. In practice it is usually unnecessary to convert all of our observations; only those of interest need be converted. These converted observations are called *z* **scores,** standard scores, or standard normal deviants. Equation 4.4 transforms any variable into its corresponding *z* score.

$$z = \frac{x - \mu}{\sigma} \tag{4.4}$$

What might not be immediately apparent here is that a *z* score is how far from the mean, in terms of standard deviations, an observation lies. An observation with a *z* score of +1 is one standard deviation greater than the mean, and an observation with a *z* score of −1 is one standard deviation less than the mean. An observation with a z score of 0 has the same value as the mean. Thus, any variant is expressed not in its actual value but in how far, in terms of standard deviations, it lies from the mean. Example 4.6 is not typical of the types of problems that biologists often deal with, but this example is very useful since much of statistical inference follows similar procedures and since it provides experience in manipulating the standard normal distribution and other probability distributions.

EXAMPLE 4.6   An Approximately Normally Distributed Variable

The height (in centimeters) of a large group ($n = 414$) of female general biology students was determined. We will consider this group to be the entire population in which we have an interest. The mean height of this group was 166.8 cm, and the standard deviation was 6.4 cm.   ■

Height in humans is an approximately normally distributed variable. We will use the standard normal distribution to answer several questions about this population.

Question 1. What is the z score of an individual who is 170 cm tall?

$$z = \frac{x - \mu}{\sigma} = \frac{170 - 166.8}{6.4} = 0.5$$

It is easy enough to comprehend that this person is 3.2 cm taller than the average student in this population, so why is it of interest to us that she is 0.5 standard deviations taller than the average? Let us ask another question.

Question 2. What proportion of the population is as short as or shorter than this 170 cm tall person? A somewhat different way of asking this same question is this: what is the probability that an individual sampled at random from this population will be 170 cm or shorter? Keep in mind in this and subsequent discussions that the area of a probability distribution corresponding to a designated proportion of the distribution may also be thought of as a probability. To solve this problem, we need to become acquainted with table A.1. When considering the use of table A.1 in this example, it will help to refer frequently to figure 4.9.

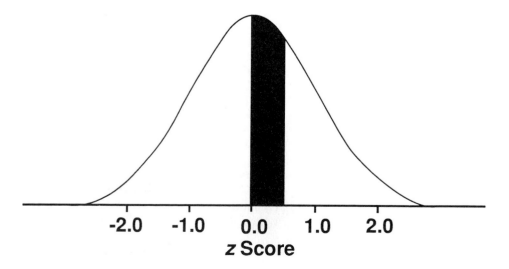

Figure 4.9
The standard normal distribution (for example 4.6, question 2).

Zero on the x-axis of this graph represents a z score of 0, which is the population mean. The shaded area of the curve (the area between the mean and our z score) represents the proportion of the standard normal distribution that falls between the mean and the indicated value of z, and these are the entries in table A.1. The left column of the table gives z scores to one significant digit. The top row extends this to 2 significant digits. For example, if we wish to know the proportion of the curve that lies between the mean and a z score of 1.23, we look down the left column to $z = 1.2$ and go across to the column headed .03 (thus, 1.23). The value we find there is 0.3907. Look this up yourself in appendix A right now. Let us return to the original question: what proportion of the standard normal distribution lies between the mean and a z score of 0.5? According to table A.1, 0.1915 (verify this for yourself). Therefore, 0.1915 (or 19%) of the individuals in this population lie between 170 cm (our person with a z score of 0.5) and 166.8 cm, which is the mean. Note that the standard normal distribution is perfectly symmetrical and that 0.5000 of the area lies above the mean and 0.5000 of the area lies below the mean. Our original question was: what proportion of the population is as short as or shorter than 170 cm? We know that 0.5000 (50%) lies below the mean (by definition). We also know that 0.1915 (19%) lies between the mean and a z score of 0.5 (corresponding to 170 cm). Therefore, 0.5000 + 0.1915, or 0.6915 (roughly 69%), lies below a z score of 0.5. We conclude that the proportion of the individuals in this population who are 170 cm or shorter is 0.6915, or in other words, approximately 69% of the individuals in this population are as short as or shorter than this individual who is 170 cm tall. This may also be interpreted to mean that the probability that any individual sampled from this population will be 170 cm or shorter is 0.6915.

You may be curious about why the 0.5000 of the standard normal curve that lies between the mean and negative infinity is not already added to the entries in table A.1. Another question might help to clarify this.

Question 3. What proportion of this population would be expected to be 163.6 cm or shorter? The z score for this observation is:

$$z = \frac{163.6 - 166.8}{6.4} = -0.5$$

Graphically, the problem looks like figure 4.10. We are trying to determine how much (what proportion) of the standard normal distribution lies to the left of (below) our z score of -0.5. Now since the standard normal distribution is symmetrical, the same proportion lies between the mean and a z score of -0.5 that lies between the mean and a z score of $+0.5$, which we already know is 0.1915. (If you do not remember how we already know this, refer back to the last question.)

Thus, the proportion that lies below a z score of -0.5 is:

$$0.5000 - 0.1915 = 0.3085$$

We conclude that approximately 31% of this population will be as short as or shorter than 163.6 cm, or that the probability that any individual sampled at random from the population will be 163.6 cm or shorter is 0.3085.

Question 4. What proportion of the population lies between 160 cm and 170 cm? This problem is shown graphically in figure 4.11. To solve it we first determine what proportion of the curve lies between the mean and 160 cm, which is:

$$z = \frac{160 - 166.8}{6.4} = -1.063$$

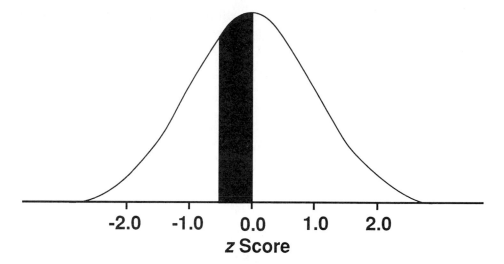

Figure 4.10
The standard normal distribution (for example 4.6, question 3).

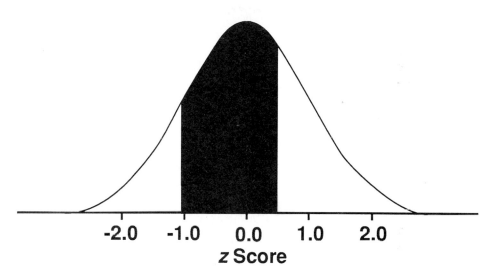

Figure 4.11
The standard normal distribution (for example 4.6, question 4).

According to table A.1, 0.3554 of the standard normal curve lies between the mean and a z score of -1.063 (-1.06, actually, since the table only goes to 2 places for z scores). Next we determine how much of the curve lies between the mean of 170 cm, for which the z score is:

$$z = \frac{170 - 166.8}{6.4} = 0.50$$

Again, according to table A.1, 0.1915 of the standard normal distribution lies between the mean and a z score of 0.50. Thus, the proportion lying between 160 cm and 170 cm, or between a z score of -1.06 and $+0.05$, is $0.3554 + 0.1915$, or 0.5469. Thus, approximately 55% of this population is expected to consist of individuals whose height is between 160 cm and 170 cm. The probability that any individual sampled at random from this population will be between 160 cm and 170 cm is 0.5469.

Question 5. What range of heights includes 0.95 (95%) of this population? This problem is somewhat different from the previous ones. Here we know the proportion of the standard normal distribution in which we have an interest (that is, we know what the z score is, and we must find the value of x

that corresponds to this z score). Table A.1 shows that 0.475 of the standard normal distribution lies between the mean and a z score of 1.96, and therefore, 0.475 lies between the mean and a z score of -1.96. Thus, 0.95 is between the mean and a z score of ± 1.96. (Refer to figure 4.8 if you need to visualize this situation.) Now since

$$z = \frac{x - \mu}{\sigma}$$

it follows that

$$x = z\sigma + \mu$$

Accordingly, the height (x) that includes 0.475 of the standard normal distribution below the mean is

$$x = (-1.96 \times 6.4) + 166.8 = 154.23$$

and the height (x) that includes 0.475 of the standard normal distribution above the mean is

$$x = (1.96 \times 6.4) + 166.8 = 179.34$$

We conclude that 95% of the individuals in this population are between the heights of 154.23 cm and 179.34 cm. Or, thinking of probabilities, there is a probability of 0.95 that any individual sampled at random from this population will be between 154.23 cm and 179.34 cm, and a probability of 0.05 that any individual sampled at random from this population will be taller than 179.34 cm or shorter than 154.23 cm.

Since we rarely know the population mean and standard deviation of a population, of what use is the information that we have been considering? From an applied standpoint, not much. However, an understanding of—or at least a speaking acquaintance with—these concepts gives one the proper frame of mind to become acquainted with another group of probability distributions, called sampling distributions, and with the underlying concepts of statistical inference.

Testing for Normality

Many of the statistical tests that we will consider in the following chapters are based on the assumption that the variable in question is at least approximately normally distributed. Fortunately, the normal distribution describes, or at least approximates, a large number of biological variables. However, one should never assume that a variable is approximately normally distributed unless there is some reason to believe that this is the case. Example 4.6 asserted that height in humans is an approximately normally distributed variable. How do we know this? One way is to examine the frequency distribution of the variable from a large sample.

Consider the male heights given in exercise 2.1. The histogram for these data, using a class interval of 5 cm, is shown in figure 4.12. Note that in general, this histogram is more or less bell-shaped, and its overall appearance is much like that of a normal distribution. For many applications this would provide sufficient justification for assuming that the distribution is approximately normal, particularly if we were using a large sample (see chapter 5 to find out why this is so).

A **cumulative frequency distribution** is somewhat easier to compare with a normal distribution, and we will digress at this point to see what this means in practical terms. If, in figure 4.12, we would add to each size class

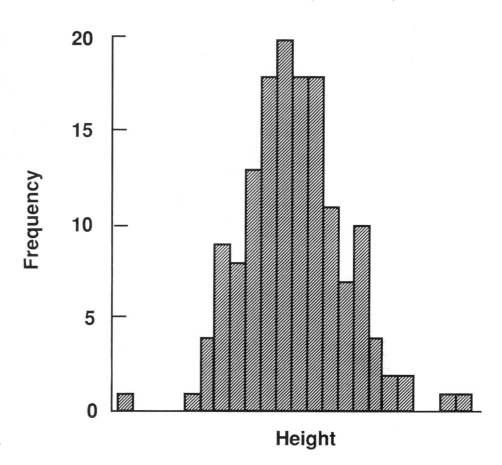

Figure 4.12
Frequency distribution of male
heights (data from exercise 2.1).

the frequency of all smaller size classes, each bar in the histogram would then represent the frequency of individuals in that size class and all smaller size classes. Accordingly, the bar representing the largest size class should equal the total number of observations in the sample. Figure 4.13 is the cumulative distribution histogram for this sample. Note that the y-axis is given as percent of the sample rather than as absolute frequencies; also note that the largest size class has a frequency of 100%. This simply means that 100% of the individuals are as short as or shorter than the tallest individual. Note also that the overall shape of the curve is roughly sigmoidal, as it should be for a normal cumulative distribution. This sigmoidal shape (more or less the shape of the letter s) is easier to discern when the distribution is plotted as a frequency polygon rather than as a histogram, as shown in figure 4.14. Again, this would be sufficient cause to assume that the distribution is approximately normal.

There is still a better way. Suppose we graphed each individual observation, rather than each size class, as a cumulative distribution. The shortest male in our sample is 161 cm and represents $\frac{1}{148}$, or 0.68%, of the total sample. The next individual is 169 cm, and combined with the one shorter individual, makes up $\frac{2}{148}$, or 1.35%, of the sample. The third individual is 170 cm tall, and with the 2 shorter individuals, represents $\frac{3}{148}$, or 2.03%, of the sample. There are 3 individuals who are 171 cm, who, combined with the three shorter individuals, represent $\frac{6}{148}$, or 4.05%, of the population. This process is continued for each observation. The tallest individual(s) should represent 100% of the sample.

The next step is to compute the cumulative normal probability distribution for a population with the same mean and standard deviation as the sample (which, for a large sample, are close approximations of the population

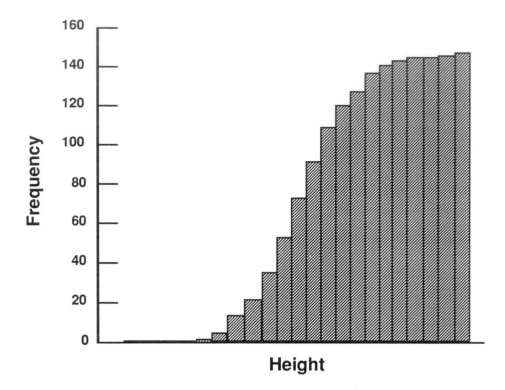

Figure 4.13
Cumulative frequency
distribution of male heights
(data from exercise 2.1).

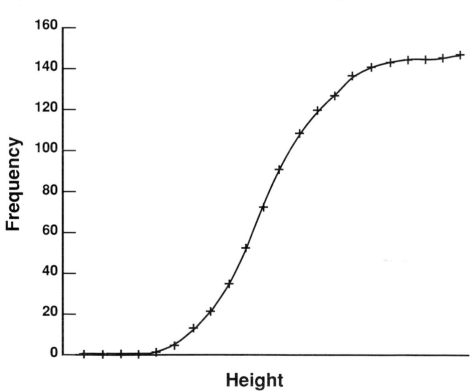

Figure 4.14
Data from figure 4.13 plotted as
a frequency polygon.

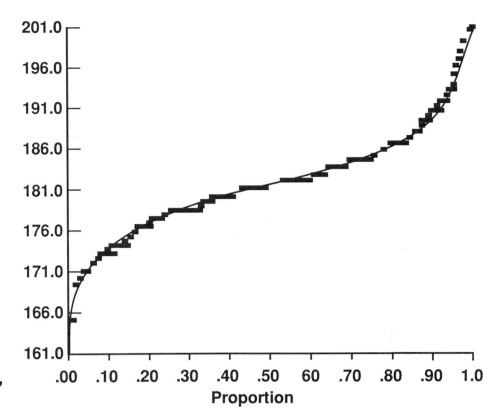

Figure 4.15
Cumulative frequency distribution of male heights (stepped line) and normal distribution of the same mean and standard deviation (smooth line) (data from exercise 2.1).

mean and standard deviation) using the same procedure that was used in the female height example discussed previously (i.e., determine what proportion of the population is expected to be 170 cm or shorter, what proportion is expected to be 171 cm or shorter, and so on).

If this strikes you as a very tedious process and hardly worth the trouble, then you are a reasonable person. However, computers hardly ever become bored with such tasks. Figure 4.15 is the computer printout of the cumulative distribution of the 148 male heights superimposed on a normal distribution of the same mean and standard deviation. Note that the two lines coincide remarkably well, and we may feel confident that height in humans, at least in males, is approximately normally distributed.

All the methods discussed thus far for determining if a variable is approximately normally distributed are graphic and depend to a large extent on the eye of the beholder. There are, of course, more analytical methods and methods that are appropriate for smaller samples. These are described in chapter 9.

Normal Approximation of the Binomial Distribution

When the number of cases, *k,* in a binomial distribution is fairly large, and *p* is not too near zero or one, the binomial distribution becomes approximately a normal distribution. How large is "fairly large"? As a rule of thumb, if the values

$$k \times p \text{ and } k \times q$$

are both equal to or larger than 5, the normal approximation is considered to be fairly accurate.

EXAMPLE 4.7

Suppose that 25 individuals are sampled from a population in which the ratio of females to males is known to be 1:1, and we wish to know the probability of obtaining a sample of 8 *or fewer* males in this sample of 25 individuals. Let p = the probability that any individual sampled will be a male (0.5), let q = the probability that any individual sampled will be a female (0.5), and let x = the number of males in which we have an interest (8 or fewer, in this case). ■

The values of $k \times p$ and $k \times q$ are both greater than 5, so we feel comfortable in approximating this binomial distribution by use of the normal distribution. The mean of a binomial variable is given by

$$\mu = kp \qquad (4.5)$$

which, for the example, is

$$\mu = 25 \times 0.5 = 12.5$$

or 12.5 males in 25 individuals.

The standard deviation is given by

$$\sigma = \sqrt{kpq} \qquad (4.6)$$

which, for the example, is

$$\sigma = \sqrt{25 \times 0.5 \times 0.5} = 2.5$$

We may regard the possible outcomes of the various combinations (no males and 25 females, 1 male and 24 females, and so on) as a normally distributed variable with a mean of 12.5 and a standard deviation of 2.5. Reference to figure 4.16 might help in visualizing this situation. The bars in figure 4.16 represent the binomial probability distribution for this example. Note that the general shape of this distribution is very similar to that of a normal distribution except that it is a bar graph. Equation 4.5 is used to compute the z score for a value of 8, given that the mean is 12.5 and the standard deviation is 2.5.

$$z = \frac{x - \mu}{\sigma}$$

The value 8 has a z score of

$$z = \frac{8 - 12.5}{2.5} = -1.80$$

In table A.1 we find that 0.4641 of the normal curve lies between the mean and $z = 1.80$ (and therefore, that 0.4641 lies between the mean and -1.80). Since 0.500 lies above the mean, the region lying beyond a z score of -1.80 is

$$0.5000 - 0.4641 = 0.0359$$

In other words, the probability of obtaining a sample of 25 individuals in which there are 8 or fewer males is 0.0359.

To calculate a z score for any outcome of a binomial distribution, equation 4.7 may be used.

$$z = \frac{x - kp}{\sqrt{kpq}} \qquad (4.7)$$

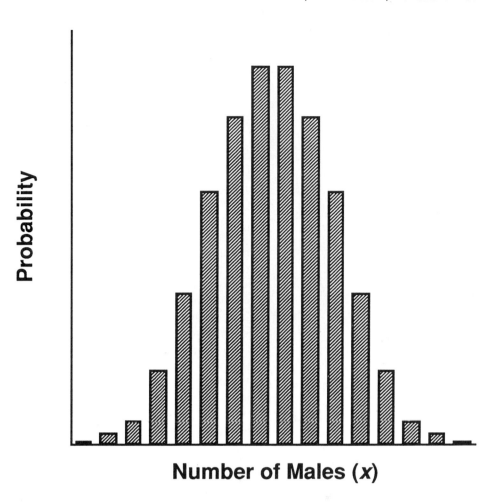

Figure 4.16
Binomial probability
distribution for k = 25 *and*
p = 0.5.

Number of Males (x)

where x is the number of cases in one category, whose probability is p; kp is the mean of a binomial variable; and $\sqrt{kpq}$ is its standard deviation. This technique provides only an approximation of the binomial probability distribution, since the binomial distribution deals with discrete variables and the normal distribution deals with continuous variables. The discrepancy between the two is not large when k is large (30 or so), but it may become appreciable when k is smaller.

Discrete Variables and the Normal Distribution

An assumption of many statistical tests is that the variable in question has an at least approximately normal distribution. Since the normal distribution is a continuous probability distribution, a question that arises (or should arise) is: is it appropriate to apply such a test to a discrete variable? As we saw in the preceding section, a discrete variable such as a binomial variable may be approximated by the normal distribution when k (the number of cases or trials) is fairly large. This also holds true for a number of discrete variables. For example, the numbers of grapes in clusters varies from a few to almost 100. A variable such as this, although it is a discrete variable, might be approximately normally distributed in the same way that a binomial variable with a large k is approximately normally distributed, and no serious harm is done when a statistical test that assumes approximate normality is used—provided, of course, that the other assumptions of the test are satisfied.

When the number of values that a discrete variable may assume is small, its distribution is very unlikely to be even approximately normally distributed, and the use of a statistical test that assumes approximate normality with such a variable is to be discouraged.

PARAMETRIC AND NONPARAMETRIC STATISTICS

Many of the most commonly used statistical tests are based on some important assumptions about the nature of the variable in question. These are that the variable is approximately normally distributed, that the variable is continuous (or if it is discrete, that it at least approximates a normal distribution), and that the variable is measured on an interval or ratio scale. When the data meet these basic assumptions, one may usually apply one of a group of tests known as **parametric tests.** When the data do not meet one or more of these assumptions, a parametric test should not be used. However, one of another group of tests called **nonparametric tests** might be appropriate. Nonparametric methods are sometimes called distribution-free methods because they make no assumption about the distribution of the variable in question. Nonparametric tests are also useful for data measured on an ordinal (ranking) scale.

In the chapters that follow, we will explore the statistical analysis of some of the more common situations encountered in biological research. In each case a parametric test will be presented along with its nonparametric counterpart, when one is available. You are encouraged to pay particular attention to both the parametric and nonparametric alternatives and to the conditions under which each is to be used.

KEY TERMS

binomial distribution
cumulative distribution
nonparametric tests
normal distribution
parametric tests

Poisson distribution
probability
   distribution
standard normal
   distribution
z scores

EXERCISES

(Exercises preceded by an asterisk are suitable for a computer solution.)

4.1 In the toss of 2 coins, what is the probability of obtaining 2 heads?

4.2 In the toss of 2 coins, what is the probability of obtaining 2 tails?

4.3 In the toss of 2 coins, what is the probability of obtaining 1 head and 1 tail?

4.4 In the toss of 6 coins, what is the probability of obtaining 2 heads and 4 tails?

4.5 In the toss of 6 coins, what is the probability of obtaining 2 or fewer tails?

4.6 In the toss of 5 dice, what is the probability of obtaining 3 twos?

4.7 In the toss of 7 dice, what is the probability of obtaining at least 2 ones?

4.8 In the toss of 7 dice, what is the probability of obtaining not more than 2 ones?

4.9 Assume that the probability that any child born in a population will be a boy is 0.5 and the probability that it will be a girl is also 0.5. For a randomly selected family of 6 children, what is the probability that there will be exactly 3 boys and 3 girls?

4.10 For the situation in exercise 4.9, what is the probability that there will be 2 or fewer girls?

4.11 For the situation in exercise 4.9, what is the probability that there will be exactly 6 boys?

4.12 For the situation in exercise 4.9, what is the probability that there will be exactly 6 girls?

4.13 In couples where each person is heterozygous for the sickle-cell gene, there is a probability of 0.25 that any child of the couple will actually have the disease, and a probability of 0.75 that any child will not have the disease. For a population of families of 6 children in which both parents are heterozygotes, what is the probability that in a randomly selected family, none of the 6 children will have the disease?

4.14 For the situation in exercise 4.13, compute the probability that exactly 3 children will have the disease.

4.15 For the situation in exercise 4.13, compute the probability that 3 or fewer children will have the disease.

4.16 For the situation in exercise 4.13, compute the probability that all 6 children will have the disease.

4.17 Construct a bar graph of the probabilities of all possible outcomes of the situation in exercise 4.13 (no children have the disease, 1 child has the disease, 2 children have the disease, and so on).

4.18 The proportion of male births to female births in a population is 49:51. Thus, the probability that any individual born into this population will be a male is 0.49 ($\frac{49}{100}$). In 1,000 families, each with 10 offspring, compute the expected frequency of families in which all 10 offspring are male.

4.19 For the situation in exercise 4.18, compute the expected frequency of families in which at least 3 offspring are males.

4.20 For the situation in exercise 4.18, compute the expected frequency of families in which there are 3 or fewer female offspring.

4.21 For the situation in exercise 4.18, compute the expected frequency of families in which there are exactly 5 male and 5 female offspring.

4.22 For the situation in exercise 4.18, compute the expected frequency of families in which all 10 offspring are females.

4.23 Construct a bar graph representing all possible expected frequencies for the situation in exercise 4.18.

4.24 Using the data from exercise 2.3 (see chapter 2), compute the Poisson probabilities and expected frequencies for $x = 0$ to $x = 8$ for a population whose mean is the same as this sample mean. Save your results for later use.

4.25 Construct a bar graph of the expected frequencies and observed frequencies for the data from exercise 2.3. Save your results for later use.

4.26   Using the data from exercise 2.3, compute the probability that a quadrate sampled at random in this population will contain exactly 12 ant lion pits.

4.27   Using the data from exercise 2.3, compute the probability that a quadrate sampled at random in this population will contain more than 7 ant lion pits.

4.28   Using the data from exercise 2.4, compute the Poisson probabilities and expected frequencies for $x = 0$ to $x = 8$ for a population whose mean is the same as this sample mean. Save your results for later use.

4.29   Construct a bar graph of the expected frequencies and observed frequencies for the data from exercise 2.4. Save your results for later use.

4.30   Using the data from exercise 2.4, compute the probability that a leaf sampled at random in this population will contain exactly 8 larvae.

4.31   Using the data from exercise 2.4, compute the probability that a leaf sampled at random in this population will contain more than 7 larvae.

4.32   In a culture containing 3×10^7 bacterial cells and 5×10^7 bacteriophage, what proportion of the bacterial cells would be expected to have no phage particles adsorbed to their cell walls? What proportion would be expected to have 5 phage particles adsorbed to their cell walls?

4.33   In a culture containing 5×10^8 bacterial cells and 3×10^8 bacteriophage, what proportion of the bacterial cells would have 3 or more phage particles adsorbed to their cell walls?

4.34   For the situation in exercise 4.32, compute the probability of x phage per cell for $x = 0$ to $x = 5$. Construct a bar graph of this distribution.

4.35   For the situation in exercise 4.33, compute the probability of x phage per cell for $x = 0$ to $x = 5$. Construct a bar graph of this distribution.
For exercises 4.36 through 4.39, regard the female mosquito fish in table B.2 (see appendix B) to be the entire population of interest. The mean length of this population is 34.29 mm and the standard deviation is 5.49 mm.

4.36   What is the probability that any individual selected at random from this population would have a length of 50 cm or larger?

4.37   What is the probability that any individual selected at random would have a length of 25 cm or shorter?

4.38   What is the probability that any individual selected at random would have a total length of between 30 mm and 40 mm?

4.39   Determine what lengths include 95% (0.95) of the population.
For exercises 4.40 through 4.43, consider the bluegills in table B.1 to be the entire population of interest. The mean standard length of this population is 152.09 mm and the standard deviation is 19.62 mm.

4.40   What is the probability that any individual sampled at random from this population will have a standard length of 170 mm or longer?

4.41   What is the probability that any individual sampled at random will have a standard length of 130 mm or shorter?

4.42   What is the probability that any individual sampled at random will have a standard length of between 148 mm and 160 mm?

4.43 What lengths include 95% (0.95) of the population?

A population of red-bellied snakes is known to have a ratio of grey color morph to red color morph of 53:47. Use the normal approximation of the binomial distribution to solve exercises 4.44 through 4.49.

4.44 What is the probability of selecting from this population a random sample of 25 snakes containing 10 or fewer grey morph individuals?

4.45 What is the probability of selecting a random sample of 25 snakes containing 4 or fewer grey morph individuals?

4.46 What is the probability of selecting a random sample of 30 snakes containing 15 or fewer grey morph individuals?

4.47 What is the probability of selecting a random sample of 20 snakes containing 3 or fewer red morph individuals?

4.48 What is the probability of selecting a random sample of 50 snakes containing between 20 and 30 red morph individuals?

4.49 What is the probability of selecting a random sample of 40 snakes containing between 15 and 30 grey morph individuals?

*4.50 Using the data from table B.2, construct a frequency distribution histogram and a cumulative frequency distribution histogram of female mosquito fish length. Use this information and any other procedures that your specific computer program has to decide if this variable is approximately normally distributed.

An Introduction to Statistical Inference

One of the most important uses biologists make of statistics is to make conclusions about populations based on samples taken from those populations. This activity is generally called **statistical inference.** There are 2 broad categories of statistical inference, illustrated by the following examples.

EXAMPLE 5.1 Estimating a Population Parameter

A random sample of 10 bluegill sunfish standard lengths was selected from table B.1. The mean of this sample was 159.40. We would like to know how well our sample mean estimates the population mean. ∎

EXAMPLE 5.2 Testing a Statistical Hypothesis

Vitamin Y is an essential nutrient, but too much of it in the diet is harmful. Accordingly, the FDA sets standards for the vitamin Y content of vitamin pills: they must contain an average of 100 units of the vitamin per pill. The manufacturer of vitamin pills assigns a biochemist skilled in statistical inference to monitor the vitamin Y content of their product. She selects a random sample of 100 pills from a particular lot and finds that their mean vitamin Y content is 100.5 units, with a standard deviation of 2.19 units. She must decide if it is reasonable that a sample with a mean of 100.5 could have been drawn from a population with a mean of 100. ∎

In example 5.1 our interest is in gaining some idea about how well our sample mean, $\bar{x}$, called a point estimator, actually estimates the population mean, μ. This general category of statistical inference is called **estimation.** In example 5.2 a hypothesis must be tested: that the average vitamin Y content of the manufacturer's pills is 100. Searching out answers to questions of this nature is generally called **statistical hypothesis testing.**

In this chapter we will deal with estimating means of populations from samples, and we will consider some important concepts of statistical hypothesis testing, using a test concerning a single population mean.

ESTIMATING A POPULATION MEAN: THE CENTRAL LIMIT THEOREM

Consider example 5.1—the mean of this sample is 159.40. Based on this sample, we would like to conclude something about the population mean. Before this can be done, however, we must consider yet another type of probability distribution, called a **sampling distribution.**

When a random sample is taken from a population, the sample that was drawn was only one of a very large number of samples of the same size that could have been taken. In fact, if we were to take repeated random samples of the same size from a normally distributed population, as illustrated in figure 5.1, and compute the mean of each sample, we would find that not only are these means likely to be different from each other but that they would have a range of values tending to cluster about some central value. In other words, these means would have a mean and standard deviation of their own and would exhibit all of the characteristics of a normally distributed random variable in

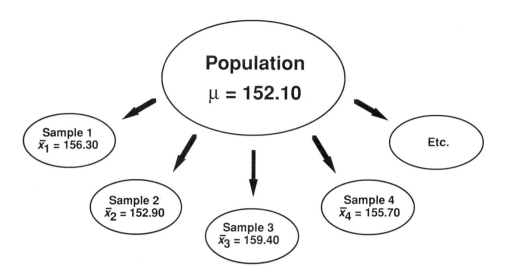

Figure 5.1
Graphic representation of
repeated samples from a
population—in this case,
repeated sample means of the
length of bluegill sunfish (data
from table B.1).

exactly the same way that observations from a normally distributed population do. It is completely appropriate to think of a sample mean as an individual observation taken from a large population of possible sample means. The probability distribution that describes the behavior of a repeated sample statistic (mean, standard deviation, and so on) is called a sampling distribution. In the case of sample means taken from a normally distributed population with a known population standard deviation, the sampling distribution is the normal distribution. This seemingly simple concept is fundamental to much of statistical inference and may be stated formally as follows.

The Central Limit Theorem

The means of samples from a normally distributed population have a normal distribution, regardless of sample size (n).

The means of samples from a population with a nonnormal distribution have an approximately normal distribution if the sample size is large (greater than 30).

The central limit theorem means, in effect, that we may assign a *z* score to a sample mean if we know (or can specify or are willing to assume) the population mean (μ) and standard deviation (σ) of the population from which our sample was taken. Recall that *z*, a variant of the standard normal distribution, for a single observation is:

$$z = \frac{x - \mu}{\sigma}$$

(5.1)

The useful thing about the central limit theorem is that we do not have to repeatedly take samples from a population to know how the means of such samples would behave if we did; they would have a normal distribution. Thus, we may consider a single sample mean from a normally distributed population (or from a nonnormally distributed population, if our sample size is large) as one of many such possible means whose distribution would be normal.

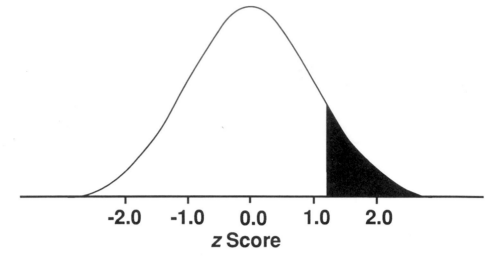

Figure 5.2
The standard normal
distribution. Shaded area is the
proportion above a z score of
1.18.

EXAMPLE 5.3

Assume that the bluegill sunfish whose lengths are given in table B.1 are the entire population of interest. The population mean length for this population is 152.10 mm, and the population standard deviation is 19.64 mm. Assume also that we have taken a random sample of 10 individuals from this population and obtained a sample mean of 159.40 mm.   ■

We may now ask this question: What is the probability of obtaining a sample mean of 159.40 mm or larger from a population whose population mean is 152.10 mm and whose population standard deviation is 19.64 mm? We may answer this question in much the same way that we answered questions about the height of women students in example 4.6 (see chapter 4)— that is, by assigning a z score to this sample mean. This problem is illustrated graphically in figure 5.2. The z score for a sample mean is given by

$$z = \frac{\bar{x} - \mu}{\sigma_{\bar{x}}} \tag{5.2}$$

The new term in this equation, $\sigma_{\bar{x}}$, is the standard deviation of our theoretical population of sample means; it is called the **standard error of the mean,** and it is calculated by

$$\sigma_{\bar{x}} = \frac{\sigma}{\sqrt{n}} \tag{5.3}$$

where σ is the population standard deviation and n is the sample size in question. For the example

$$\sigma_{\bar{x}} = \frac{19.64}{\sqrt{10}} = 6.21$$

The z score for our sample is therefore

$$z = \frac{159.40 - 152.10}{6.21} = 1.18$$

We could, of course, calculate this more simply by combining equations 5.2 and 5.3 to give

$$z = \frac{\bar{x} - \mu}{\dfrac{\sigma}{\sqrt{n}}} \tag{5.4}$$

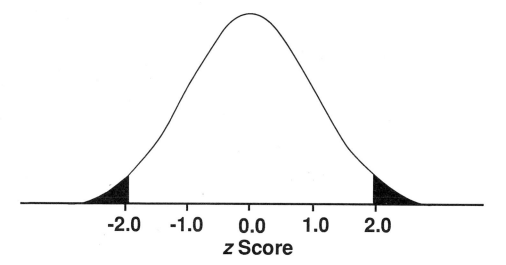

Figure 5.3
The standard normal
distribution. Shaded areas
represent 0.05 of the
distribution.

Consulting table A.1 we find that 0.3810 of the standard normal distribution lies between the mean and a *z* score of 1.18. Subtracting this value from 0.5000 gives 0.1190 of the standard normal distribution that lies above a *z* score of 1.18 (the shaded portion of figure 5.2). Thus, the probability of drawing a sample of 10 individuals with a mean as high as or higher than 159.40 mm is 0.1190. Another way of saying this is that approximately 12% (0.1190 $\times$ 100) of all of the samples of 10 that might possibly be drawn from this population would have a mean of 159.40 or higher.

There is another question we might ask, and one that is more to the point: Within what range would we expect 95% of the sample means of samples of 10 to lie? This is equivalent to the question asked in example 4.6 regarding the range of heights that would include 95% of the population of female freshman biology students. Refer to figure 5.3. We are looking for those values of sample means that include the unshaded portion of this curve, or the values

$$\mu + z_{(0.475)}\sigma_{\bar{x}} \tag{5.5}$$

and

$$\mu - z_{(0.475)}\sigma_{\bar{x}} \tag{5.6}$$

(Recall that 0.95 of the standard normal distribution lies between *z* scores of -1.96 and 1.96.) For the example these values are

$$152.10 + (1.96 \times 6.21) = 164.27$$

and

$$152.10 - (1.96 \times 6.21) = 139.93$$

Thus, 95% of the samples of 10 that we might draw from this population would have a sample mean between 139.93 and 164.27. Note that the sample mean we obtained for this example, 159.40, is within this range. Another way of thinking about this is as follows: there is a probability of 0.95 that any sample of 10 we might draw from this population would have a sample mean between 139.93 and 164.27 (conversely, there is a probability of 0.05 that any sample mean would lie outside of this range—either smaller than 139.93 or larger than 164.27).

Confidence Interval of μ When σ is Known

The information we have just considered is not of very much practical use, since we would hardly want to estimate a population mean from a sample mean when we already know the value of the population mean. However, the concepts we have just examined provide the basis for a good deal of statistical inference, and it is important to grasp these concepts. To see a practical application of this information, we will change our assumptions about example 5.1 slightly. Suppose we do not know the population mean of this population *19.64* but we do know the population standard deviation: ~~6.21~~. (Exactly how we might know this is not important. The wonderful thing about imaginary situations is that one may imagine anything that suits the purpose at hand.) Using the sample mean, we can calculate a range of values within which we have a specified level of confidence that the population mean lies. This range is called a **confidence interval** of the mean. The procedure we will follow in this case is applicable when the population standard deviation (σ) is known or can be assumed to have a particular value.

Assumptions of the Test

1. The sample is a random sample from the population of interest.
2. Measurement is on an interval or ratio scale, and the variable is continuous. (If the variable is discrete, it may assume a wide range of values—see chapter 4.)
3. The variable is approximately normally distributed.
4. The population standard deviation is known.

Using $\overline{x}$ as a point estimate of μ and armed with a knowledge of the population standard deviation, the upper limit (UL) and lower limit (LL) for a 95% confidence interval of the mean are given by

$$UL_{0.95} = \overline{x} + (1.96 \times \sigma_{\overline{x}}) \qquad (5.7)$$

and

$$LL_{0.95} = \overline{x} - (1.96 \times \sigma_{\overline{x}}) \qquad (5.8)$$

For the example

$$UL_{0.95} = 159.40 + (1.96 \times 6.21) = 171.57$$

and

$$LL_{0.95} = 159.40 - (1.96 \times 6.21) = 147.23$$

Or we may combine these two expressions and write

$$147.23 < \mu < 171.57$$

or simply

$$\mu = \overline{x} \pm 12.17$$

Thus, we feel 95% confident that the population mean of this population is included by the interval 147.23 to 171.57. (It is. Remember that we actually know the population mean of this population to be 152.10, but for this illustration we are assuming that it is unknown.) Another way of saying this is that there is a 95% (0.95) probability that this range includes the population mean. To calculate a 99% rather than a 95% confidence interval for a mean, one simply uses 2.576 as the appropriate value for z, since this is the z score that defines 99% (0.99) of the standard normal distribution—see table A.1.

CAUTION

When thinking about a confidence interval of a mean, or any other parameter, it is incorrect to conclude that there is a 95% (or 99% or whatever) probability that the parameter lies between the upper and lower limits. The parameter has a fixed value, usually unknown to us, and therefore there is no probability associated with it: it is whatever it is. The probability in such a case is that our confidence interval includes (or "encloses") the parameter in question.

Confidence Interval of μ When σ is Unknown: The t Distribution

In real life we usually have no knowledge of the population standard deviation; instead we must rely on the sample standard deviation as a point estimate of the parameter. Given a large sample from a normally distributed population, no serious error is committed by using the sample standard error as an estimate of the population standard error and using the standard normal distribution to compute confidence limits for a mean, although it is not strictly correct to do so. When the population standard deviation is unknown, the sampling distribution of means departs somewhat from normality, and this departure becomes larger as sample size becomes smaller. There is, however, a sampling distribution that better describes the distribution of means when the sample standard deviation must be used. This is the t distribution, or as it is sometimes known, Student's t distribution.

Student's t distribution is very similar to the normal distribution in most respects, except that it is defined by the degrees of freedom ($n - 1$) in addition to the mean and standard deviation. Recall that the proportion of the standard normal distribution that occurs between the mean and any z score may be determined by reference to table A.1. We may also determine the value of z that includes a specified proportion of the standard normal distribution by using table A.1. For example, a z value of ± 1.96 includes 0.95 (or excludes 0.05) of the standard normal distribution.

When considering the distribution of sample means, it is useful to think of t as having the same general properties as z, except that the values of t that exclude a given proportion of the t distribution vary with sample size. We may determine the value of $\pm t$ that excludes certain specified proportions of the t distribution by reference to table A.2.

Suppose we wish to determine what value of t excludes 0.05 of the t distribution with 4 degrees of freedom. Figure 5.4 is a graphic representation of table A.2. The shaded portion of the curve is the proportion that lies outside of plus or minus any particular value of t. Keep this in mind while referring to table A.2. The column headings are the proportion indicated by the shaded areas in figure 5.4. Note that the proportions of the t distribution given in table A.2 and figure 5.4 include both "tails" of the distribution. This is an important distinction between table A.1, the normal distribution, and table A.2. The left column ("df") in table A.2 indicates degrees of freedom (remember that the t distribution is partially determined by degrees of freedom). The numbers in the body of the table are values of t that correspond to a designated proportion

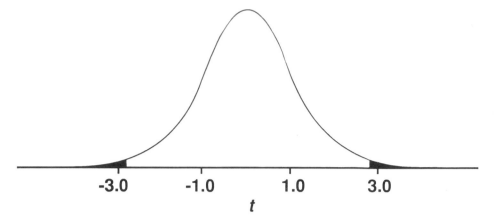

Figure 5.4
A t distribution with 4 degrees of
freedom. Shaded areas represent
0.05 of the distribution, with
0.025 in each tail.

of the distribution for the specified degrees of freedom. In the present case, the number corresponding to 0.05 and 4 degrees of freedom is 2.776, which is found in the table by following the 0.05 column down and the 4 df row across (refer to table A.2 now). Thus, ±2.776 is the value of *t* that excludes 0.05 of the *t* distribution (or includes 0.95). This is shown graphically in figure 5.4.

Suppose we wish to determine the value of *t* that excludes only the upper 0.05 of the *t* distribution with 4 degrees of freedom. Table A.2 gives *t* values that exclude a certain proportion of the distribution equally divided between both tails, as shown in figure 5.4. Thus one-half of the indicated proportion is in the upper tail of the curve, and one-half is in the lower tail of the curve. Therefore, when we are interested in only one tail, we simply double the proportion indicated in table A.2. For this problem we consult table A.2 for 4 degrees of freedom and a probability (proportion) of 0.10 (rather than 0.05), where we find that 2.132 is the *t* value that excludes the upper 0.05 of the *t* distribution. This is shown graphically in figure 5.5.

Note in table A.2 that *t* for any particular proportion of the *t* distribution becomes smaller as the degrees of freedom becomes larger. At infinite degrees of freedom (sample size of infinity plus one?) the value of *t* that excludes 0.05 of the distribution is 1.960—exactly the value of *z* that excludes 0.05 of the standard normal distribution. The reason for this is that as the degrees of freedom increase, the *t* distribution tends to become a normal distribution.

Returning now to our original purpose—determining the confidence interval for a mean when we must use the sample standard deviation—we use the *t* distribution rather than the normal distribution as the appropriate sampling distribution.

EXAMPLE 5.4

A random sample of 20 male mosquito fish was collected, and total length (in millimeters) was determined. The sample mean length ($\bar{x}$) was 21.0 mm, and the sample standard deviation (*s*) was 1.76 mm. We wish to construct a 95% confidence interval for the population mean. Length in male mosquito fish is known to be approximately normally distributed. ∎

This is a fairly typical situation. Both the mean and the standard deviation of the population must be estimated from their sample values, and the sample size is fairly small. The assumptions of the test are essentially the same as those for the construction of the confidence interval of a mean when the population standard deviation is known. They are repeated here.

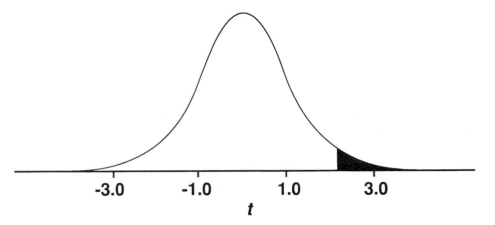

Figure 5.5
A t *distribution with 4 degrees of freedom. Shaded area represents 0.05 of the distribution in one tail. Compare with figure 5.4.*

Assumptions of the Test

1. The sample is a random sample from the population of interest.
2. Measurement is on an interval or ratio scale, and the variable is continuous. (If the variable is discrete, it may assume a wide range of values—see chapter 4.)
3. The variable is approximately normally distributed (see chapter 4).

The upper limit for a 95% confidence interval is given by

$$\text{UL}_{0.95} = \bar{x} + (t_{(0.05,\ n-1)}) \times s_{\bar{x}} \tag{5.9}$$

and the lower limit is given by

$$\text{LL}_{0.95} = \bar{x} - (t_{(0.05,\ n-1)}) \times s_{\bar{x}} \tag{5.10}$$

where $t_{(0.05,\ n-1)}$ is the tabular value of t at $n-1$ degrees of freedom, which delineates 0.95 of the t distribution (found in table A.2 in the column headed "0.05" and the row corresponding to the appropriate degrees of freedom), and $s_{\bar{x}}$ is the sample standard error, $(\frac{s}{\sqrt{n}})$. For the example

$$\text{UL}_{0.95} = 21.0 + (2.093 \times 0.394) = 21.825$$

and

$$\text{LL}_{0.95} = 21.0 - (2.093 \times 0.394) = 20.175$$

or

$$20.175 < \mu < 21.825$$

or

$$\mu = \bar{x} \pm 0.825$$

Thus, we conclude there is a 95% (0.95) probability that the range of 20.175 mm to 21.825 mm includes the population mean.

STATISTICAL HYPOTHESIS TESTING AND THE SCIENTIFIC METHOD

Science and the scientific method have been defined in many different ways. A definition I have always liked, although it is a bit restrictive and excludes some of the things we call "science," goes something like this: science is an organized body of knowledge about the physical universe, obtained by observation and experiment and used to make generalizations (theories) about the nature of the physical universe. There are some very important concepts embedded within this short definition, including why we need to use statistics!

Science begins with observations, which are simply events in the physical universe that we may detect in some way. Recall from chapter 2 that we referred to a measurement of a single individual in a population as an "observation" and designated its value as x. Observations are fine, but they tend to not be very useful in and of themselves. It is when we try to explain the observations that science begins. A tentative explanation of one or more observations is called a hypothesis, and a good hypothesis has the following attributes.

Attributes of a Scientific Hypothesis

1. It is consistent with the observations, which is to say that if it is correct, it will explain what has been observed.
2. If it is false, it can be shown to be false. In other words, it can be tested. The test of a hypothesis is called an experiment.

Note that we do not say that if a hypothesis is true it can be shown to be true. Rather, we say that if it is false it can be shown to be false. Why such a negative attitude? Philosophers of science tell us that a false hypothesis may be proven to be false but a true hypothesis may not be proven to be true! Accordingly, a hypothesis is considered to be true when, by experiment (testing), it is not possible to prove that it is false.

When efforts to prove a hypothesis false (experiments) fail to do so, our confidence in the correctness of the hypothesis increases. If the hypothesis has general or widespread application to events in the physical universe, we designate it as a theory. Like a hypothesis, a true theory cannot be proven to be true, but a false theory can be proven to be false. Lamarck's theory of the inheritance of acquired characteristics was a pretty good theory for its time—it simply failed to stand up to repeated testing (experiment), and so it was abandoned in favor of a better theory.

It has been said that science does not proceed by proving things—it proceeds by disproving things—and eventually, incorrect theories will be proven to be incorrect. This business of attempting to disprove hypotheses and theories is what we call the scientific method. It operates by an *if . . . then* logic. *If* the hypothesis (theory) is correct, *then* this will be the outcome of the experiment. If the outcome of the experiment is something other than what the hypothesis (theory) predicts, then we reject the hypothesis and look for a better explanation. This process is often called hypothesis testing, and it is the activity that distinguishes science from other forms of human activity.

Testing the conclusion(s) of a research endeavor by statistical means—what we usually call statistical inference or statistical hypothesis testing—is a special application of the scientific method. It is often possible, particularly in statistical hypothesis testing, to state a question or hypothesis in such a way that there are only 2 possible outcomes. These are "A is true" and "A is not true." Suppose that, unknown to us, the first of these statements, "A is true," is correct. We could not prove this statement directly if in fact it is correct because, as you will recall, a true hypothesis cannot be shown to be true. Suppose, though, that we tested the statement "A is false" and proved it to be incorrect (a false hypothesis can be shown to be false). If the statement "A is false" is disproved, and the statement "A is true" is the only other alternative, then we are left to conclude that the statement "A is true" is in fact correct!

Unfortunately, things are hardly ever this simple. When we must rely on a sample of individuals from a larger population to obtain information about that population, there is always a probability that our sample is not really representative of the population. However, using statistical hypothesis testing, we can specify a probability that our conclusion is incorrect. If this probability is low (by long-standing tradition, 0.05 or less), we feel confident that our conclusion is correct.

In statistical hypothesis testing, we usually attempt to reduce the question at hand to 2 choices, much like the "A is true" and "A is not true" dichotomy discussed previously, and to specify exactly what we mean by these 2 choices. Only one of these statements is tested, as before, and its parameter of interest is specified. The choice tested is called the **null hypothesis,** usually symbolized by H_0, and the alternative is called the research hypothesis, or simply the **alternative hypothesis,** symbolized as H_1.

An understanding of the nature of the null hypothesis is critical to the understanding of the nature of statistical hypothesis testing. Essentially, it is the hypothesis of no difference. (Null, as an adjective, means, among other things, "amounting to nothing" or "having zero magnitude." It is derived from the Old French term *nul,* meaning "none.") Note carefully in the following examples that the null hypothesis always contains an equal sign, or at least an implied equal sign.

Test of a Hypothesis Concerning a Single Population Mean: The One Sample *t*-Test

Example 5.2 should help to clarify the concepts discussed above, and it will serve to introduce a few new ones. It might be useful to review the normal distribution (chapter 4) and the *t* distribution in conjunction with this example. Refer back to example 5.2 on p. 64 now.

In this case the population mean (μ) is known; it is 100 units. We know this because of the specified FDA requirement. In this situation there is a null hypothesis to be tested: that the mean vitamin Y content of the pills is 100 units, or

$$H_0: \mu = 100 \text{ units}$$

Note the equal sign in this expression. The alternative hypothesis (the one that is true if the null hypothesis is false) is

$$H_1: \mu \neq 100 \text{ units}$$

We assume, for the moment, that the population mean of our hypothetical population of vitamin pills is 100 units. We do not know if this is true; it is the population mean specified by the null hypothesis, and we wish to determine if it might be true. If we conclude that it is not true, then we conclude that the only other possibility—the alternative hypothesis—is true.

Recall from the discussion of sampling distributions of means that there is a certain probability that a sample with a mean of 100.5 units could be drawn from a population with a population mean of 100 units by chance. Remember, we do not know the population mean. However *if* it is 100, *then* there is a certain probability associated with drawing a sample with a mean that differs by as much as 0.5 units from the population mean of 100. The value

$$t = \frac{\overline{x} - \mu}{s_{\overline{x}}}$$
(5.11)

for repeated samples from a population has a *t* distribution. When the computed value of *t* is equal to or greater than the tabular value of *t* for a specified area of the *t* distribution (usually 0.05 or 0.01), we reject the null hypothesis, since the probability of obtaining such a value of *t* when the null hypothesis is true is quite small (0.05 or less, or 0.01 or less).

The assumptions of this test are the same as those for computing a confidence interval using the *t* distribution (refer back to p. 71).

For the example

$$t = \frac{100.5 - 100}{0.219} = 2.283$$

The tabular value of *t* for $p = 0.05$ and 99 degrees of freedom (we use 100 degrees of freedom, since 99 is not tabulated) is 1.984 (see table A.2). Therefore, we may reject H_0.

This problem is shown graphically in figure 5.6. The *x*-axis represents the distribution of *t* that would be expected under the null hypothesis. The values $+1.984$ and -1.984 delimit 0.95 of the distribution. Thus, there is a probability of 0.95 that any sample we might take from this population would have a *t* value of between -1.984 and $+1.984$, and a probability of 0.05 that any sample would have a value lower than -1.984 or greater than $+1.984$. Since our value of 2.283 is very unlikely if the null hypothesis is true, we reject the null hypothesis and conclude that the alternative hypothesis is true. We are 95% confident that we have reached the correct decision. Refer to figure 5.6 once again. The shaded areas—the proportion of the curve beyond ± 1.984—are sometimes referred to as the region of rejection because when the calculated value of *t*, the **test statistic,** falls within this region, the null hypothesis is rejected. (A test statistic is a calculated value, such as *t*, whose distribution is known when the null hypothesis is true.) It is rejected because, if it were true, we would expect, with a probability of 0.95, to obtain a calculated value of *t* that falls within the unshaded portion of figure 5.6.

There are 2 explanations for obtaining a *t* value as high as we did in this example. One is that the null hypothesis is true, and the sample mean we obtained differed from the population mean by as much as it did by chance alone. In other words, we obtained a very unlikely sample! The second explanation is that the null hypothesis is false. Since the probability of drawing a sample with a mean that differs this much from the population mean by chance alone is very small (less than 0.05), we conclude that the null hypothesis is false. As we will see in the next section, this conclusion could be incorrect.

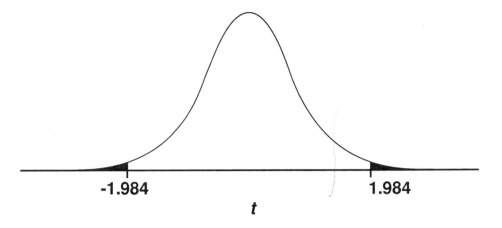

Figure 5.6
A t distribution with 99 degrees of freedom for a two-tailed probability, $\alpha = 0.05$.

As previously stated, H_0 is usually rejected when the probability that a sample value (such as a sample mean) would be obtained from a population with a population value (a mean, for example) specified by the null hypothesis is equal to or smaller than some predetermined level, such as 0.05 or 0.01. This value is referred to as alpha (α). Note that alpha is not an exact probability associated with a particular value of the test statistic but rather a predetermined probability at or below which we conclude that the null hypothesis is false.

Ideally, the researcher determines what level of alpha he or she will regard as sufficient for rejecting H_0 before the experiment is conducted. In the real world, however, an alpha level of 0.05 is usually regarded as sufficient for rejecting a null hypothesis. Note that in the example above, the calculated value of t (2.283) was considerably larger than the **critical value** of t (the value that delimits the specified area of the distribution). Thus, we know that if the null hypothesis is true, the probability of obtaining a t value with an absolute value as large as or larger than the value we obtained is actually less than 0.05. Table A.2 allows us to find a range for this probability, but not its exact value, since this table specifies values of t for only certain probabilities. Consulting table A.2 at 100 degrees of freedom gives the critical value for a probability of 0.05 as 1.984, which is smaller than our calculated value of t (2.283), and a critical value of 2.364 for a probability of 0.02, which is larger than our value of t. Thus, the actual probability associated with our value of 2.283 lies between 0.05 and 0.02, or

$$0.02 < p < 0.05$$

In this expression p is the probability of obtaining a value of t as great as or greater than the value that was obtained (2.283, for this example) if the null hypothesis is true. This is usually referred to as the **p value.** For the example the p value lies somewhere between 0.02 and 0.05, as determined by use of table A.2. Most statistical packages for computers give exact p values. For this example the p value is 0.025, as determined by computer. When the p value is equal to or lower than a predetermined value of alpha, usually 0.05 but occasionally 0.01, the null hypothesis is rejected. In this case, had we chosen to select an alpha level of 0.01, we would not reject the null hypothesis. Who or what determines the alpha level? We will explore this question in the next section.

Note that in this example we have included one-half of alpha, ($\frac{\alpha}{2} = 0.025$) in each tail of the distribution (figure 5.6). This is because the null hypothesis specified that $\mu = 100$, and if rejected, it would tell us only that $\mu \neq 100$. Thus, we would reject H_0 if t fell in either the upper or the lower tail of the distribution (i.e., $t \leq -1.984$, or $t \geq 1.984$). This is called a two-tailed test. Obviously, in two-tailed tests the absolute value of t is of interest.

In some situations we have an interest in only one tail of a distribution, and these are referred to as one-tailed tests. This can be illustrated by changing our example slightly. Suppose the FDA requirement for vitamin pills specifies that pills must contain an average of at least 100 units of vitamin Y per pill. They may contain 100 units or more, but they may not contain less than 100 units. The null hypothesis for this case is

$$H_0: \mu \geq 100$$

and the alternative hypothesis is

$$H_1: \mu < 100$$

(Note that the null hypothesis contains an equal sign.)

In this situation our interest is only in the lower tail of the t distribution. The shaded portion of figure 5.7 represents 0.05 of the t distribution when our interest is only in the lower tail, and the value of t that delimits this area is -1.660. This is found in table A.2 by looking in the column headed ''0.1'' at 100 degrees of freedom. (Table A.2 gives only two-tailed probabilities. To find a one-tailed probability, we must consult the column for twice the desired probability.) Thus, a t value of -1.660 or lower would be justification for rejecting the null hypothesis. Since our calculated value for t is much higher than this, we cannot reject H_0. We conclude that the vitamin pills contain 100 or more units of Y per pill. Note that this one-tailed test does not permit us to conclude that the pills contain exactly 100 units or more than 100 units; it only indicates that they do not contain less than 100 units. Note also that in a one-tailed test, the sign of t is of importance.

The same procedure is used when we wish to conduct a one-tailed test with alpha only in the upper tail of the distribution. In this case the null hypothesis would be that the pills contain not more than 100 units, or H_0: $\mu \leq 100$, and the alternative hypothesis is $H_1: \mu > 100$. In this case the critical value of t is $+1.660$, and we would reject H_0 when our calculated value of t is equal to or greater than this value. For the example we may reject H_0 and conclude that the pills contain more than 100 units. This situation is shown in figure 5.8.

How does one know when a one-tailed test is appropriate and when a two-tailed test is appropriate? That depends on the null hypothesis, which in turn depends on the question we wish to answer. The 3 questions we asked concerning the vitamin pill example are fairly typical (although vitamin Y is an imaginary nutrient). If we wish to know if the vitamin content of the pills is either more than or less than 100 units, a two-tailed test is indicated. On the other hand, if interest centers only in determining if the content is more than 100 units, we would choose a one-tailed test. Note, however, that we would not reject H_0 if the content of the pills was less than 100 units. Thus, it is very important to state the null hypothesis in such a way that, if it is rejected, we will arrive at a sensible answer to the research question we had in mind.

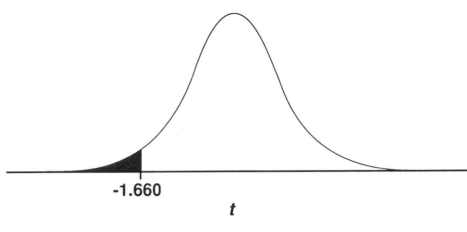

Figure 5.7
A t distribution with 99 degrees of freedom for a lower one-tailed probability, α = 0.05.

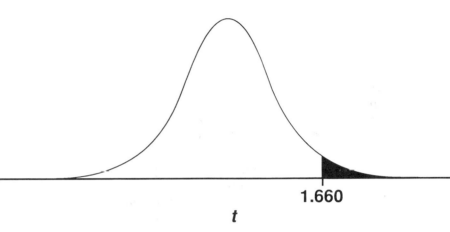

Figure 5.8
A t distribution with 99 degrees of freedom for an upper one-tailed probability, α = 0.05.

Statistical Decision-Making

Ideally, the researcher sets alpha before the statistical analysis is done—usually at either 0.05 or 0.01. In example 5.2 our biochemist (or the FDA) set alpha at 0.05. Since the calculated value of *t* was greater than the critical (table) value for *t,* she rejected H_0. The actual probability associated with the calculated value of *t* (the *p* value) in this case was 0.025, as determined by computer, or between 0.02 and 0.05, as determined from table A.2. In either case $p \le 0.05$, so H_0 was rejected. Suppose, however, that she had been willing to reject H_0 only if $p \le 0.01$ (i.e., she had set alpha as 0.01). In this case she would have been unable to reject H_0! So what is the truth of the matter? Is H_0 true or false? The fact that it is possible to reach 2 contradictory conclusions from the same data, depending on where we set alpha, should convince you that there is always an element of subjectivity involved in statistical inference. In fact, our biochemist cannot know with absolute certainty if the vitamin pills do or do not contain an average of 100 units of vitamin Y unless she analyzes every pill (i.e., the entire population), in which case there would be no pills left to sell!

You may have realized by now that there is a possibility of reaching an incorrect conclusion when that conclusion is based on a statistical test. This is indeed the case. In fact, 2 types of errors are possible in such a situation.

In example 5.2 suppose the null hypothesis was actually true—that the average vitamin content of the pills was in fact 100 units—but the statistical test indicated otherwise. Remember in this instance there is a probability of 0.05 or less of obtaining a t value of 2.283 or even more extreme when H_0 is true. This probability is so low that we would be "safest" in rejecting the null hypothesis. Such an error—rejecting the null hypothesis when it is in fact true—is called a **type I error.** The probability computed in a statistical test, which is 0.025 (or 0.05 or less, in this example), is the probability of making a type I error. The risk that such an error will occur is sometimes called the **alpha risk,** and we compute its probability when we test a statistical hypothesis.

But there is another possible error—failing to reject a null hypothesis when in fact it is false. This is called a **type II error,** and its probability, called beta (β), is usually not calculated (although it can be, using methods we will not discuss here). The risk of making a type II error is sometimes called the **beta risk.**

Table 5.1, sometimes called a "truth table," illustrates the relationship between the null hypothesis and the type I and type II errors.

Table 5.1 The Possible Consequences of a Statistical Decision

		H_0 True	H_0 False
	Fail to Reject H_0	Correct	Type II Error
Decision			
	Reject H_0	Type I Error	Correct

Important points about alpha and beta that you might wish to keep in mind are as follows.

1. Alpha, as previously stated, is fixed by the investigator and/or the scientific community at a certain level, usually 0.05 (or sometimes 0.01). Therefore, its value is known. If the probability associated with our test is equal to or smaller than alpha, the null hypothesis is rejected. Beta, on the other hand, is usually not calculated, and therefore its value is usually not known. For any given test, beta decreases as sample size increases. Thus, large samples result in a smaller beta risk than do smaller samples for any particular test. Beta increases as the sample mean comes closer to the null hypothesis. In example 5.2 the null hypothesis specified a mean of 100, while the sample mean was 100.5. Thus, in this situation there is a fairly large beta risk. Had the sample mean been 110 or some such value, the beta risk would be much lower.

2. The beta risk varies among statistical tests. In some it is higher, while in others it is lower. A test with a low beta risk is said to be powerful. Thus, some tests are more powerful than others. Accordingly, when one has a choice of two or more tests for testing the same null hypothesis, the most powerful test should always be used.

3. Designating a lower level for alpha obviously decreases the risk of a type I error, but at the same time it increases the risk of a type II error. Suppose that in our vitamin pill example, the null hypothesis of 100 units per pill is actually false. Using an alpha level of 0.05 leads to the correct conclusion. However, if alpha were set at 0.01, the null hypothesis would not be rejected, resulting in a type II error. One reason alpha is so frequently set at 0.05 is that this level represents a fairly reasonable compromise between the type I error and the type II error.

You have no doubt heard or read of results of a statistical test as being referred to by its **significance level**—that is, as being "significant" or perhaps even "highly significant." In the context of the previous discussion of alpha and beta, "significant" usually means that H_0 may be rejected at an alpha level of 0.05 (i.e., when the p value associated with the test statistic is 0.05 or less). Such a conclusion is sometimes said to be "significant at the 95% level." "Highly significant" usually means that H_0 may be rejected when alpha is set at 0.01—sometimes stated as "significant at the 99% level."

This particular terminology is most unfortunate, since most people who use the English language understand (correctly) that "significant" means approximately the same thing as "important," "meaningful," or "of some consequence." Thus, when some scientist informs you that his or her results are "highly significant," try not to be overly impressed! This simply means that he or she has very likely reached the proper conclusion about a question that might be important or that might be totally trivial.

Fortunately, this particular terminology, and even the use of predetermined alpha levels, seems to be losing popularity in favor of simply expressing the p value associated with the test statistic. Thus, in example 5.2 our biochemist might report that H_0 was rejected at $p = 0.025$ (or $0.02 < p < 0.05$, if she used table A.2 rather than a computer) instead of reporting that the difference in vitamin content between her company's pills and the FDA requirement was "significant, but not highly significant" (which, of course, a normal person would interpret as "important, but not very important"). There are actually several ways that results of a statistical test might be reported, and you will encounter all of these in the biological literature. All mean more or less the same thing. Using example 5.2, these are as follows.

"The result is significant at the 95% level."

"The result is significant." By implication this means the same thing as the first statement.

"$p \leq 0.05$." This tells the reader that the p value associated with the test statistic was equal to or less than 0.05, but there is no indication of how much less. The reader is free to decide for himself or herself if H_0 should be rejected.

"$0.02 < p < 0.05$." This tells the reader that the p value of the test was less than 0.05 but not as small as 0.02. This method of reporting is even better than the immediately preceding example, since it gives the reader a much better indication of the actual p value.

"$p = 0.025$." This statement tells the reader that the probability associated with the test statistic is 0.025 and lets the reader share with the investigator the decision about whether or not to reject H_0. The disadvantage of this particular choice is that most statistical tables do not give exact probabilities. However, most computer programs for statistics do give these exact probabilities. With the general availability of personal computers and statistical software, this method of reporting results is gaining popularity.

Of these various ways of reporting the same result, the last one has much to recommend it. Not only does it avoid the use of words such as "significant" and "highly significant," which have unwanted, misleading, and unavoidable connotations, but it also lets the consumer of scientific information decide what level of alpha is acceptable to him or her.

Reporting a Sample Mean

How should one report a sample mean in a scientific presentation? There are several more or less conventional ways of doing this, depending on the information one wishes to convey. The information in example 5.2 might be reported in any one of the following ways.

1. The mean plus or minus the standard deviation ($\overline{x} \pm s$), which for example 5.2 is 100.5 ± 2.19. While this tells the reader something about the variation of the measured variable in the population, it provides little information about how well the sample mean estimates the population mean, unless the reader wishes to calculate a confidence interval for himself or herself.
2. The mean plus or minus the standard error ($\overline{x} \pm s_{\overline{x}}$). This is perhaps the most common way of reporting a sample mean, and it does provide a rough idea of how well the sample mean estimates the population mean. However, it does not give this information as precisely as does a confidence interval.
3. The mean plus or minus the 95% (or 99%) confidence interval, or $\overline{x} \pm CI_{(0.95)}$. This method of reporting a sample mean has a great deal to recommend it. The information conveyed is directly accessible to the reader and is not misleading.

Sample means are often represented graphically, using one of the 3 methods just discussed. Such a graph is shown in figure 5.9. The points on the graph represent sample means, and the vertical lines, sometimes called "error bars," represent plus or minus one standard deviation, one or two standard errors, or a confidence interval. Again, by convention the error bars usually represent $\pm s_{\overline{x}}$. A common (but mistaken) belief is that if these error bars of 2 or more means do not overlap, then the differences between these means are "significant." This is not necessarily true (see chapter 7), so the use of $\overline{x} \pm s_{\overline{x}}$ either graphically or in written form, is often misleading.

Steps in Testing a Statistical Hypothesis

Most statistical hypothesis testing more or less follows a particular sequence of steps. In solving the exercises at the end of this and subsequent chapters, you might find it useful to follow this sequence.

1. State, very clearly, the question you are attempting to answer.
2. Identify the characteristics of the sample and the variable in question. Is the scale of measurement nominal, ordinal, ratio, or interval? Is the variable known to be (or may it be assumed to be) approximately normally distributed? If not, what is the distribution?
3. What sampling distribution describes a sample of this kind, and what is the appropriate statistical test?
4. Based on your answers to numbers 1, 2, and 3 above, state the null hypothesis and the alternative hypothesis. Is a one-tailed or a two-tailed test appropriate? Determine the level of alpha at or below which you will reject the null hypothesis. (This is sometimes referred to as the decision rule.)
5. Make the appropriate calculation. If the probability of obtaining this calculated value is equal to or smaller than the preselected value of alpha, reject the null hypothesis and accept the alternative hypothesis.

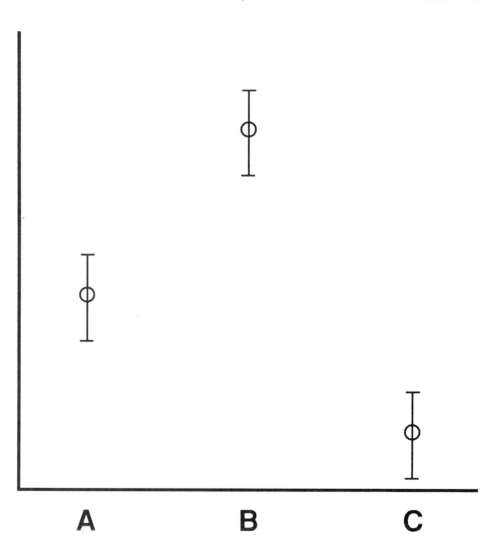

Figure 5.9
Graphic representation
of sample means.

KEY TERMS

alpha risk
alternative hypothesis
beta risk
confidence interval
critical value
estimation
null hypothesis
p value
sampling distribution

significance level
standard error of the
  mean
statistical hypothesis
  testing
statistical inference
test statistic
type I error
type II error

EXERCISES

5.1   Compute the 95% confidence interval for the samples of 10, 20, and 30 bluegill sunfish standard lengths that you obtained in exercise 1.1 (see chapter 1). In this case assume the population standard deviation is known (41.95 mm) but the population mean is unknown.

5.2 Compute the 95% confidence intervals for the samples of 10, 20, and 30 male mosquito fish lengths that you obtained from exercise 1.2. Assume the population standard deviation is known (2.64 mm) but the population mean is unknown.

5.3 Compute the 95% confidence intervals for the samples of 10, 20, and 30 female mosquito fish lengths that you obtained from exercise 1.3. Assume the population standard deviation is known (5.49 mm) but the population mean is unknown.

5.4 Compute the 95% confidence intervals for the samples of 10, 20, and 30 resting pulse rates that you obtained from exercise 1.4. Assume the population standard deviation is known (13.51 bpm) but the population mean is unknown.

5.5 Compute the 95% confidence intervals for the samples of 10, 20, and 30 reaction times from exercise 1.5. Assume the population standard deviation is known (40.43 msec) but the population mean is unknown.

5.6 Combine your results from any of exercises 5.1 through 5.5 with those of your classmates. Construct a graph like that shown in figure 5.9 for samples of 10, another graph for samples of 20, and yet a third graph for samples of 30, plotting the means and confidence intervals of your sample and of those of your classmates on the y-axis and the "sample number" on the x-axis. Draw a horizontal line on this graph that represents the population mean of the population you sampled (these values are given at the end of the respective data sets in appendix B). Do all of the confidence intervals include the population mean? If not, explain why some might not.

5.7 Based on the number of students in your class, approximately how many of the confidence intervals from exercise 5.6 would you expect might not include the population mean?

5.8 Compute the 99%, 95%, and 90% confidence intervals for the population mean using the sample data from exercise 2.1 (see chapter 2). Neither the population mean nor the standard deviation are known in this case.

5.9 Compute the 99%, 95%, and 90% confidence intervals for the population mean using the data from exercise 2.2. Neither the population mean nor the standard deviation are known in this case.

5.10 Compute the 99%, 95%, and 90% confidence intervals for the population mean using the data in exercise 3.4 (see chapter 3). Neither the population mean nor the standard deviation are known in this case.

5.11 The weights (in milligrams) of spleens of 9 newly hatched turkeys are given below. Compute the 99%, 95%, and 90% confidence intervals for the population mean. (Data from F. McCorkel.)

18.9	20.4	15.9
19.9	17.4	24.0
21.3	16.2	19.3

5.12 The 72-hour blastogenesis of chicken peripheral blood lymphocytes (10^6 cells/well) are given below. Compute the 99%, 95%, and 90% confidence intervals for the population mean. (Data from F. McCorkel.)

236	314	471
305	414	616
304	414	301
225	369	402

5.13   The number of eggs produced in a single brood by 11 female green iguanas is given below. Compute the 99%, 95%, and 90% confidence intervals for the population mean. (Data from T. Miller.)

33	50	46
33	53	57
44	31	60
40	50	

5.14   The activity of o-diphenol oxidase (ulO$_2$/mgP/min) was measured in 15 tomato plants. The results are given below. Compute the 99%, 95%, and 90% confidence intervals for the population mean.

36	29	41	45	33
28	43	32	37	41
29	32	43	37	25

5.15   The snout vent length (in centimeters) in 25 newly born garter snakes selected at random from several litters are given below. Compute the 99%, 95%, and 90% confidence intervals for the population mean.

6.5	4.3	4.6	6.0	4.7
6.2	5.8	5.4	5.2	4.8
4.9	5.0	4.7	3.4	3.9
5.1	5.4	4.8	3.8	6.1
4.8	3.9	3.8	6.1	5.2

5.16   The total weight (in grams) of 14 female iguanas are given below. Compute the 99%, 95%, and 90% confidence intervals for the population mean. (Data from T. Miller.)

1450	2000	2000
1550	2435	2750
2200	1550	1800
1500	1050	2850
1650	2300	

5.17   The FDA has established that the concentration of a certain pesticide in apples may not exceed 10 ppb. A random sample of 100 apples from a major orchard had an average pesticide content of 10.03 ppb with a standard deviation of 0.12 ppb. Are the apples within the FDA requirement?

5.18   A certain enzyme in the liver of fish is considered an indicator of trace amounts of a dangerous pollutant that is difficult to detect by chemical methods. Enzyme activities of less than 50 units per gram of liver (fresh weight) are taken to indicate the presence of the pollutant. The following random sample was taken from a certain body of water and the enzyme concentrations were found to be the following.

48	43	51	42
50	42	44	45
56	49	44	47
50	49	38	46
38	52	32	56

Is this evidence that the water is polluted?

5.19   A turkey geneticist wished to select for breeding purposes hens whose eggs have an average weight of 100 grams. The mean weight of a sample of 20 eggs from one hen was 97 grams, with a standard deviation of 2.5 grams. Should this hen be kept in the breeding program?

Inferences Concerning Two Populations

One of the more commonly used groups of statistical tests are those designed to test whether 2 or more populations differ from each other in some way. We are most often interested in differences in the means of these populations, but we may also test for differences in variability or distribution. This chapter considers methods for dealing with questions about whether 2 population means differ. Chapter 7 considers procedures for testing hypotheses about more than 2 population means.

In the first part of this chapter, we will deal with methods of determining if differences in the means of 2 **independent samples** represent real differences in the 2 population means. In this context *independent* refers to the fact that the 2 samples are from different populations. In the second part of this chapter, we deal with **related samples,** or as they are often called, matched-pairs samples. In related-samples experiments, each individual is measured twice (in effect serving as its own control) or carefully matched pairs of individuals are measured.

TESTS FOR TWO POPULATION MEANS

One of the more commonly used groups of tests are those designed to test whether 2 populations have different means. When its assumptions are met, the most powerful test available is the *t*-test for independent samples. A very useful nonparametric test that is applicable in many instances when the data do not meet the assumptions of the *t*-test for independent samples is the Mann-Whitney test. Both tests are discussed in the following sections.

The *t*-Test for Independent Samples

Recall from the previous discussion of the central limit theorem (chapter 5) that the means of samples from a population of unknown variance have a *t* distribution if the measured variable is at least approximately normally distributed. We used this concept in chapter 5 to make inferences about a single population mean. By a similar line of reasoning, we may use the *t* distribution to test whether 2 population means differ from each other. The null hypothesis of such a test is that the means of the 2 populations are equal, or

$$H_0: \mu_a = \mu_b$$

If repeated sample means from a population have a *t* distribution, then it follows that the difference between repeated *pairs* of sample means taken from a population or from 2 populations with the same population mean have a *t* distribution.

$$t = \frac{(\bar{x}_a - \bar{x}_b) - (\mu_a - \mu_b)}{s_p} \tag{6.1}$$

where $(\bar{x}_a - \bar{x}_b)$ is the difference between the 2 sample means and $(\mu_a - \mu_b)$ is the difference between the 2 population means. When the null hypothesis is that the 2 population means are equal (the most common case), $(\mu_a - \mu_b)$ is zero. s_p is a standard error for the difference between means and is based on the pooled estimate of variance of the 2 samples. It is calculated as shown in equation 6.2.

> **Assumptions of the Test**
>
> 1. The 2 samples are random samples from the 2 populations of interest.
> 2. The measured variable is approximately normally distributed and is continuous. If the variable is discrete, then it may assume a large range of values (see chapter 4).
> 3. Measurement is on an interval or ratio scale.

The t-test for independent samples is both powerful (meaning that the probability of a type II error is not high) and robust (meaning that it is still valid when the characteristics of the data depart somewhat from the assumptions). However, the power of the test decreases as the distance between the data and the assumptions increases. When assumptions 2 or 3 are not met, the Mann-Whitney test, which is discussed later in this chapter, might be appropriate. To conduct the test, the test statistic t is computed by equation 6.2.

$$t = \frac{(\bar{x}_a - \bar{x}_b) - (\mu_a - \mu_b)}{\sqrt{\dfrac{s^2_a}{n_a} + \dfrac{s^2_b}{n_b}}} \qquad (6.2)$$

The degrees of freedom for this case are $n_a - 1$ or $n_b - 1$, whichever is the smaller of the two. The expression in the denominator of equation 6.2 is the standard error of the difference between the 2 means.

EXAMPLE 6.1   A t-Test

The ratio of length to width of root hair cells in two species of plants (A and B) of the same genus were measured using random samples. Assume this variable is approximately normally distributed. We wish to know if the 2 population means differ. The results were as follows.

	Species A	Species B
n	12	18
$\bar{x}$	1.28	4.43
s^2	0.112	7.072

Data from T. Ruhlman

The null hypothesis for this example is

$$H_0: \mu_A = \mu_B$$

and the alternative hypothesis is

$$H_1: \mu_A \neq \mu_B$$

Because of the way the question is stated (do the 2 population means differ?) this is a two-tailed test. Substituting the example values in equation 6.2 gives

$$t = \frac{1.28 - 4.43}{\sqrt{\dfrac{0.112}{12} + \dfrac{7.072}{18}}} = -4.967$$

Since this is a two-tailed test, we are interested only in the absolute value of our calculated t. The critical value of t for 11 degrees of freedom and $\alpha = 0.05$ is 2.201 (see table A.2). We therefore reject H_0 that the 2 population means are equal and conclude that they are not equal.

Equation 6.2 may be used when the variances of the 2 populations are not equal or when they are equal. When it is known or may be assumed that the 2 population variances are equal, a somewhat more powerful t-test may be applied using a somewhat different method of calculating the pooled estimate of variance and using $(n_A + n_B - 2)$ degrees of freedom. Since the procedures for testing equality of variance for small samples are not very powerful, many researchers prefer to use the method described here.

A Nonparametric Test for Two Independent Samples: The Mann-Whitney Test

There are a number of situations in which the data collected in an experiment do not meet the assumptions of the t-test for independent samples, which is a parametric test. For instance, measurement might be on an ordinal scale, the distribution of the variable might not be normal, or the variable might be discrete and have only a few possible values. In such cases one is well advised to use the Mann-Whitney test, which is the nonparametric counterpart of the t-test for 2 independent samples. It tests whether 2 samples could have been drawn from identical populations. Specifically, it tests whether 2 populations of the same but unspecified distribution differ with respect to central tendency (usually the median). The null hypothesis of the Mann-Whitney test is that the samples were drawn from identical populations with respect to the variable being considered. The assumptions of the test are that the 2 population distributions are of the same shape (but not necessarily normal) and that random samples have been drawn from the 2 populations. The sample sizes need not be equal.

To conduct the test, the data of the 2 samples must be ranked together (but the identity of the sample to which any datum belongs must be preserved). The lowest value in either sample receives a rank of 1, the next lowest the rank of 2, and so on. Tied scores receive the average rank that each would have, had they not been tied. It is not as complicated as it sounds. Example 6.2 will help clarify this.

EXAMPLE 6.2   The Mann-Whitney Test

Male gully cats are territorial; they hold territories up to several hectares in size. The territory size of random samples of gully cats from 2 locations were measured (in hectares) with the results shown as follows. We wish to know if there is a difference in territory size between these 2 populations.

Location A	(Rank)	Location B	(Rank)
7	1.5	21	11
21	11	29	14
17	7	32	15
7	1.5	18	8
20.6	9	35	16
24	13	36	17
14	6	37	18
21	11	10	4.5
10	4.5	8	3
		45	19
$n_a = 9$		$n_b = 10$	
$\Sigma R_a = 64.5$		$\Sigma R_b = 125.5$	

■

Why might we choose the Mann-Whitney test for these data rather than a *t*-test for independent samples? Because we suspect that territory size in these animals is not normally distributed. (Since the animal and the data are both imaginary, we may suspect whatever we wish!)

First, all of the observations in both samples are ranked, with tied observations receiving the average rank that they would have if they were not tied. Note in the "location A" sample that there are two observations of 7, and these are the lowest of all of the observations. If they are not tied, they would receive the ranks 1 and 2. However, since they are tied, they receive the average rank that they would have, or $\frac{(1+2)}{2} = 1.5$. Ranking proceeds in this manner until all observations have been ranked.

We now compute 2 values of the test statistic, *U,* by the following equations:

$$U_a = n_a n_b + \frac{n_a(n_a + 1)}{2} - \Sigma R_a \qquad (6.3)$$

where n_a and n_b are the sample sizes of samples A and B, and ΣR_a is the sum of the ranks of sample A. U_b is then calculated by

$$U_b = n_a n_b - U_a \qquad (6.4)$$

For the example

$$U_a = (9 \times 10) + \frac{9(9 + 1)}{2} - 64.5 = 70.5$$

and

$$U_b = (9 \times 10) - 70.5 = 19.5$$

Table A.4 gives the critical values of U for various levels of α when both sample sizes are smaller than 20. The null hypothesis is rejected if the *smaller* of the calculated values of U (19.5, in this example) is equal to or *smaller* than the table value at the desired level of α for a one- or two-tailed test, whichever is appropriate. In this case we are conducting a two-tailed test (why?), and we will set α at 0.05. Accordingly, the critical value of U found in table A.4 is 70. Since our smaller calculated U is smaller than this, we reject H_0.

Note that table A.4 applies only when sample sizes are 20 or less. If either sample has more than 20 observations, the probability distribution of U is normal, and the normal distribution approximation of U is given by

$$z = \frac{\left[U - \left(\frac{n_a n_b}{2} \right) \right]}{\sqrt{\frac{n_a n_b (n_a + n_b + 1)}{12}}} \tag{6.5}$$

where U is either U_a or U_b, calculated according to equations 6.3 and 6.4. H_0 is rejected at $\alpha = 0.05$ if $z \geq \pm 1.96$ for a two-tailed test.

TESTS FOR TWO RELATED SAMPLES

It is sometimes advantageous, particularly in experimental work where the choice of subjects is under the control of the investigator, to use paired, matched, or related samples rather than independent samples. In certain instances an individual may even be used as its own control, while in other instances individuals that are as nearly alike as possible may be selected to receive 2 or more different experimental treatments. One problem associated with conducting experiments is ensuring that the control group is as nearly like the experimental group as possible, except for the treatment given the experimental group. Using paired samples, it may be assumed that any difference between the groups is associated with the treatment given them.

Suppose we wish to test the effect of some drug on pulse rate in humans. We might randomly assign individuals to 2 groups and give 1 group (the control group) a placebo and the other group (the treatment group) the experimental drug. Suppose also that the individuals in our study differed with respect to age, sex, smoking, caffeine consumption, and exercise habits. This would introduce a great deal of variation among the individuals that is not related to the treatment given them. We assume that since individuals were randomly assigned to the 2 groups, the variance of the 2 groups would be equal. This variation from individual to individual that is not related to the treatment given is called **error variance.** It is discussed in more detail in chapter 7.

Recall that for a test for a difference in population means for 2 independent samples, the test statistic, t, is computed by

$$t = \frac{\overline{x}_A - \overline{x}_B}{s_p}$$

Now if the difference between the 2 population means is fairly small and the variance is large, we would run a fairly high risk of failing to reject the null hypothesis of no difference between the 2 means when in fact it is false. In other words this situation would be likely to produce a type II error. This risk could be reduced by using a very large sample, but there is a much more efficient way.

Suppose we paired or matched the subjects in the study, selecting for the pairs individuals that were as nearly alike as possible, and then we randomly assigned one member of each pair to one group (treatment or control) and the other member of the pair to the other group. Most of the variation between 2 individuals of a pair would presumably be caused by the difference in treatment given them since, in most other respects, they are alike. Thus, in a paired design, our interest focuses on the *differences* between pairs, and the tests conducted are essentially one-sample tests. This will become clear as we proceed.

The Paired *t*-Test

When measurement is on an interval or ratio scale and when the variable under study may be assumed to be approximately normally distributed, the *t*-test for paired (matched) samples may be used. This test is equivalent to the one sample *t*-test discussed in chapter 5, since, in effect, we are dealing with one sample—the difference in the observed individuals before and after some treatment, or the difference between matched pairs of individuals under different specified conditions.

Assumptions of the Test

1. Measurement is on an interval or ratio scale.
2. The distribution of the variable is approximately normal.
3. Each individual is measured twice—once before the specified treatment and again following the specified treatment—or matched pairs of individuals are measured.
4. The data constitute a random sample from the population of interest.

EXAMPLE 6.3   A Paired *t*-Test

The weights of 10 individual centim eaters were determined at one week of age and again at two weeks of age. The data are as follows.

Animal Number	Weight (in grams) at:		
	One week	Two weeks	D
1	1.0	2.5	1.5
2	1.3	2.6	1.3
3	0.9	2.5	1.6
4	0.8	2.2	1.4
5	1.1	2.6	1.5
6	1.2	1.0	−0.2
7	0.7	2.0	1.3
8	0.6	2.1	1.5
9	1.5	2.6	1.1
10	2.0	3.6	1.6
	Mean difference = $\overline{D}$ = 1.26 s = 0.536		

The null hypothesis for a two-tailed test in a case such as this is that the population mean difference ($\mu_{\overline{D}}$) in weight at weeks 1 and 2 is equal to zero, or

$$H_0: \mu_{\overline{D}} = 0$$

and the alternative hypothesis is

$$H_1: \mu_{\overline{D}} \neq 0$$

Thus, we would reject H_0 if the creatures either gained or lost weight during this one-week period. On the other hand, we might wish to use a one-tailed test in a case like this; thus, our question might be: do these creatures gain weight between 1 week and 2 weeks of age? In this case, the null hypothesis would be

$$H_0: \mu_{\overline{D}} \leq 0$$

and the alternative hypothesis would be

$$H_1: \mu_{\overline{D}} > 0$$

where $\mu_{\overline{D}}$ is the population mean difference.

In either case the test is conducted in the same way. The critical value of t is what is different. (Recall that the critical value of t for a one-tailed test when alpha is set at 0.05 is found in table A.2 in the column headed "0.1".)

Our interest here is focused on the difference in weight between one week and two weeks (the column headed "D") and the mean of these differences ($\overline{D}$), which is 1.26. This is the sample mean difference from week one to week two. The expression

$$t = \frac{\overline{D}}{s_{\overline{D}}} \tag{6.6}$$

has a t distribution with $n - 1$ degrees of freedom (n, in this case, being the number of matched pairs). $\overline{D}$ is the sample mean difference, and $s_{\overline{D}}$ is the standard error of the mean difference, calculated by

$$s_{\overline{D}} = \frac{s}{\sqrt{n}} \tag{6.7}$$

For the example

$$s_{\overline{D}} = \frac{s}{\sqrt{n}} = \frac{0.536}{\sqrt{10}} = 0.169$$

and

$$t = \frac{\overline{D}}{s_{\overline{D}}} = \frac{1.26}{0.169} = 7.46$$

As before, we consult table A.2 to determine if H_0 may be rejected. The critical value of t for 9 degrees of freedom at alpha = 0.05 is 2.262. Therefore, we reject H_0 and conclude that there is a significant weight change between weeks 1 and 2. The exact p value, determined by computer, is 0.0000385. Had we conducted this test as a one-tailed test, the critical value of t would be 1.833.

Nonparametric Tests for Two Related Samples

In matched pairs or repeated measures experiments in which the data do not satisfy the assumptions of the parametric test, perhaps because the distribution of the variable is not approximately normal or because measurement is on an ordinal scale, one of two nonparametric tests for 2 related samples may be used.

The Sign Test. The sign test is a nonparametric test for paired or matched samples that is useful when the direction ($<>$) of the difference between matched pairs can be determined but when the magnitude of the difference cannot. The null hypothesis tested is that $p(A > B) = p(A < B) = 0.5$, where

A and B are measurements of the matched pair. In plain English this means that the probability that A is greater than B is equal to the probability that A is smaller than B for any given pair.

To conduct the test, each pair is given either a plus or a minus sign, depending on which member of the pair is larger. Tied pairs (no difference) are dropped from the analysis, and n is reduced accordingly. This is essentially a binomial distribution problem in which we compare the frequency of pluses and minuses with the distribution expected under the null hypothesis

$$H_0: \text{frequency of pluses} = \text{frequency of minuses}$$

with $p = 0.5$, $q = 0.5$, and $k = $ the number of paired observations (n). This is exactly analogous to determining the probability of obtaining x heads and $k - x$ tails in k tosses of a coin.

EXAMPLE 6.4

A biological statistics class was given a test. Immediately after the test was completed, each student was asked if he or she felt better than, worse than, or the same as before he or she took the test. Nine reported feeling better, 1 reported feeling worse, and 2 reported no change. Using this sample of 12 students, we wish to know if taking tests affects how students feel.   ∎

In this situation each individual is paired with himself or herself and is in effect measured twice—feeling before the test and feeling after the test. Thus, we can detect the direction of change in any individual (better or worse), but not the magnitude of the change. The sign test is appropriate for such a situation, and it is conducted in the following manner.

Nine students reported feeling better and would receive a plus sign, while 1 reported feeling worse and would receive a minus sign. The 2 who reported no change are dropped from the sample, and the sample size is reduced accordingly. Let $x = $ the frequency of the less frequent sign (1, in this case) and $k - x = $ the frequency of the more frequent sign (9, in this case). The probability of obtaining 1 minus sign and 9 plus signs in 10 "trials" ($k = 10$) is given by the now familiar expression

$$p(x) = \frac{k!}{x!(k - x)!} p^x q^{(k - x)}$$

As before, we are interested in the probability of the exact outcome we observed plus any even more extreme outcomes (in this case 0 minuses and 10 pluses is the only more extreme outcome). For the example

$$p(1) = \frac{10!}{1! \times 9!} 0.5^1 \times 0.5^9 = 0.009760$$

and

$$p(0) = \frac{10!}{0! \times 10!} 0.5^0 \times 0.5^{10} = 0.000976$$

$$p(1) + p(0) = 0.009876 + 0.000976 = 0.010736$$

or a probability of approximately 0.011 of obtaining 1 minus value and 9 plus values or an even more extreme case if the null hypothesis is true. This is a one-tailed probability, but the way the example is phrased ("better" or "worse") indicates a two-tailed test. Thus, the probability of obtaining the observed result or one even more extreme if H_0 is true is twice the one-tailed probability, or $0.010736 \times 2 = 0.021472$. We therefore reject H_0.

Why is this a two-tailed test? Simply because we did not specify the direction of change in feeling in the null hypothesis. Had our research hypothesis been that taking biological statistics tests makes students feel better, the null hypothesis would have been that taking such tests makes students feel no different or worse. Had this been the null hypothesis, it could be rejected with a p value of 0.010736 rather than one of 0.021472.

The Wilcoxon Signed-Ranks Matched-Pairs Test. This nonparametric test is appropriate when the direction of the difference between matched pairs can be determined and when the differences can be ranked with respect to each other. Thus, it is appropriate for data measured on an ordinal scale, or for data measured on an interval or ratio scale in situations in which the variable is not normally distributed. Unlike the sign test, this test does give greater weight to pairs with larger differences than to pairs with smaller differences. The differences are ranked with respect to their absolute values (i.e., -1 has a lower value than either $+2$ or -2), but the sign of the difference is retained with the rank. As in the sign test, pairs in which there is no difference are dropped from the sample, and the sample size is reduced accordingly.

H_0 in this test is that the sum of the positive ranks in a population is equal to the sum of the negative ranks in the population.

EXAMPLE 6.5   The Wilcoxon Matched-Pairs Test

Female gully cats are thought to be more aggressive when they have young. Accordingly, aggressiveness scores on a scale of 1 to 10, with 10 being most aggressive, were obtained for a group of 7 females without young and for these same 7 females with young. The scores were as follows.

Female Number	Without Young	With Young	D	R
1	3	7	4	4
2	2	8	6	6
3	5	4	-1	$1.5(-)$
4	6	9	3	3
5	5	10	5	5
6	1	9	8	7
7	8	9	1	1.5

Note that animals 3 and 7 were tied with a rank of 1.5. The fact that animal 3 had a difference in before and after scores of -1 and animal 7 had a difference of $+1$ makes no difference with respect to their ranks. However, the fact that animal 3 had a negative score is noted. To calculate the value of the test statistic, designated as T, the sum of ranks that have a negative sign and the sum of ranks that have a positive sign are taken. T is the smaller of these 2 sums. For the example, T is 1.5. Critical values of T are given in table A.5. H_0 is rejected if the calculated value of T is equal to or *smaller* than the tabular value of T.

Table A.5 gives values of n (sample size) up to 25. For larger samples, T is approximately normally distributed and the normal distribution may be used, where

$$z = \frac{T - \dfrac{n(n + 1)}{4}}{\dfrac{n(n + 1)(2n + 1)}{24}} \tag{6.8}$$

H_0 is rejected if z is equal to or larger than plus or minus 1.96 for alpha 0.05.

COMPUTER SUPPLEMENT

Most statistical programs for computers are capable of conducting all of the tests in this chapter, although some may not do the nonparametric tests. Figure 6.1 is the MINITAB printout testing whether male and female mosquito fish are of different lengths, using the data from table B.2.

```
:MTB > twosample 'males' 'females'
:
:TWOSAMPLE T FOR males VS females
:            N       MEAN      STDEV    SE MEAN
:males      854      23.60      2.64     0.090
:females    797      34.29      5.50     0.19
:
:95 PCT CI FOR MU males - MU females: (-11.115, -10.27)
:
:TTEST MU males = MU females (VS NE): T= -49.83   P=0.0000   DF=   1126
:
:MTB >
```

Figure 6.1
MINITAB printout of a t-test for independent samples (data from table B.2).

KEY TERMS

error variance   related samples
independent samples

EXERCISES

For each of the following problems, state the appropriate null hypothesis and the alternative hypothesis, conduct the appropriate test, and state a conclusion. Reject H_0 if p ≤ 0.05. *Assume the variable in question to be approximately normally distributed unless instructed otherwise.*
(Exercises preceded by an asterisk are suitable for a computer solution.)

The *t*-Test for Independent Samples

6.1   Data on resting pulse rates were collected for random samples of 57 men and 63 women between the ages of 18 and 21. We wish to know if there is a difference in the mean pulse rate of men and women in this population. The results were as follows.

	Men	Women
$\bar{x}$	73.789	82.270
s	10.395	13.750
n	57	63

6.2 Data on reaction time (in milliseconds) for random samples of 58 men and 68 women were collected. We wish to know if there is a difference in reaction time between men and women in this population. The results were as follows.

	Men	Women
$\bar{x}$	170.21	181.31
s	32.643	45.988
n	58	68

6.3 Random samples of largemouth bass and smallmouth bass were taken from a lake, and their standard lengths (in millimeters) were determined. We wish to know if the mean standard length differs between the 2 species in this lake. The results were as follows (data from J. Kagel).

	Largemouth Bass	Smallmouth Bass
$\bar{x}$	272.8	164.8
s	96.4	40.0
n	125	97

6.4 The mass (in grams) of random samples of adult male tuatara from 2 locations are given below. We wish to know if animals from location A have a larger mean mass than animals from location B (data from J. Gillingham).

Location A		Location B
510	790	650
773	440	600
840	435	600
505	815	575
765	460	452
780	690	320
235		660

6.5 Liver alcohol dehydrogenase activity in 2 random samples of catfish was determined. One sample was taken upstream from a brewery, and the other sample was taken downstream from the brewery. We wish to know if living downstream from a brewery increases liver alcohol dehydrogenase in these animals. The results were as follows.

Upstream	Downstream
10	30
25	32
8	28
11	35
19	29
7	32
5	32
30	38
	31

6.6   The effect of copper sulfate on the mucus cells in the gill filaments of a certain species of fish was investigated. We wish to know if exposure to copper sulfate reduces the number of mucus cells in this species. The number of mucus cells per square micron in the gill filaments of untreated fish and in fish exposed for 24 hours to copper sulfate (mg/l) were as follows. We wish to know if exposure to copper sulfate affects the number of mucus cells.

Untreated	Exposed
16	10
17	8
12	10
18	12
11	13
18	14
12	6
15	5
16	7
14	5
18	10
12	11
	9
	8

6.7   Random samples of cranberries were collected from 2 bogs. We wish to know if the mean weight of cranberries (in grams) differs between the 2 bogs. The results were as follows.

	Bog A	Bog B
$\bar{x}$	1.31	1.27
s	0.25	0.27
n	25	27

6.8   Spleen weights of road warblers infected with the avian malaria parasite and of those that were parasite free were determined. We wish to know if infection by this parasite affects spleen weight in this species.

Infected	Healthy
25.6	20.8
27.8	22.9
29.3	26.0
26.9	23.2
26.0	25.1
25.9	23.7
	25.6
	23.2

6.9   A certain species of bacterium was grown with either glucose or sucrose as a carbon source. After a period of incubation, the number of cells ($\times 10^6$) was determined. Is there a difference in growth rate of the bacterium between the 2 carbon sources?

Glucose	Sucrose
6.3	5.8
5.7	6.2
6.8	6.0
6.1	5.1
5.2	5.8

6.10   Six randomly selected pea plants were treated with a plant growth regulator, and 6 randomly selected plants were not treated. We wish to know if the growth regulator affects internode growth.

Internode Length (in millimeters) in	
Treated Plants	Untreated Plants
15.2	13.5
12.3	9.8
11.6	10.2
14.8	8.7
10.0	9.2
14.2	9.0

6.11   Growth of pine seedlings in a chemically defined liquid substrate with and without molybdenum was measured. We wish to know if growth is greater in the presence of molybdenum.

Growth (centimeters/year)	
Without Molybdenum	With Molybdenum
3.2	4.5
4.5	6.2
3.8	5.8
4.0	6.0
3.7	7.1
3.2	6.8
4.1	7.2

6.12 The surface pH of 2 lakes was measured at several randomly selected sites in each lake. We wish to know if the hydrogen-ion concentration of the 2 lakes is different. (Caution: pH is not a linear measurement! The data should be converted to hydrogen-ion concentrations.)

Lake A	Lake B
7.1	6.9
7.2	6.8
6.9	6.7
7.0	6.8
7.1	7.0

6.13 The soil pH in a coniferous forest and in a deciduous forest was measured at several randomly selected places in each site. We wish to know if the hydrogen-ion concentration is different in the 2 sites. (Caution: pH is not a linear measurement! The data should be converted to hydrogen-ion concentrations.)

Coniferous	Deciduous
5.9	6.2
6.0	6.4
6.2	6.1
5.8	6.3
5.6	6.4
5.7	6.0
5.8	6.2
5.7	5.9
5.6	6.1
5.9	6.0

*6.14 Using the data in table B.3 (see appendix B), determine if male athletes have faster reaction times than male nonathletes.

*6.15 Using the data in table B.3, determine if women smokers have faster pulse rates than women nonsmokers.

*6.16 Using the data in table B.2, select random samples of 30 male mosquito fish and 30 female mosquito fish. From these samples determine if the population mean length for females is greater than the population mean length for males.

The Mann-Whitney Test

6.17 Do people find hairy spiders scarier than nonhairy spiders? To find out, 20 people were randomly assigned to 2 groups of 10 each. One group viewed a hairy spider, and the other group viewed a very similar but nonhairy spider. Each person was asked to rate the spider she or he viewed on a scariness scale from 1 to 10 (10 being most scary). The results were as follows.

Hairy		Nonhairy	
10	10	7	5
8	9	6	4
7	9	8	5
9	5	6	6
9	8	1	3

6.18 Male hoop snakes, upon encountering one another, may engage in a protracted ritualized combat behavior until one establishes himself as dominant over the other. We would like to know if these encounters last longer in the presence of a female. Twenty-four males were randomly assigned to pairs. Six randomly selected pairs were tested in the presence of a female, and 6 were tested in the absence of a female. This variable is not known to be approximately normally distributed; in fact, it probably is not. The results were as follows.

Interaction Time (in minutes)	
Pairs without Female	Pairs with Female
10	59
15	35
8	70
30	65
1	43
80	90

6.19 The 72-hour blastogenesis of chicken peripheral blood lymphocytes from a group treated with PHA and from an untreated group are given below. This variable is *not* approximately normally distributed. We wish to know if treatment with PHA has an effect on blastogenesis of these cells.

Control	Treated
1631	87700
50102	69553
1369	76215
41188	366
387	40104
498	38661
259	141153
329	154805
4330	123075
5002	627
658	126175
300	11223
	300

6.20 Seven tomato plants were treated with chlorogenic acid to determine if this would influence the activity of the enzyme *o*-diphenol oxidase in the leaves. A control group of 7 plants were not treated. We do not know if this variable is approximately normally distributed, nor is it possible to determine this with a sample as small as this. Does this treatment affect activity of the enzyme?

Treated	Untreated
35	10
45	18
36	8
11	29
41	17
29	8
38	11

6.21   Aerial surveys of several randomly selected areas of forest land were used to determine damage by a certain insect. Some areas had been sprayed several years before the survey to control the insect and some had never been sprayed. A scale of 1 to 10 was used to assess damage, with 10 being most severe. We wish to know if there is a difference in previously sprayed areas and in areas that had never been sprayed.

Sprayed Areas	Unsprayed Areas
3	2
0	5
1	6
5	3
2	3
1	4
5	8
3	2
6	1
0	8
	2
	6
	5

6.22   Assume that in exercise 6.4 the variable is not approximately normally distributed. Conduct the appropriate test, and state your conclusions.

The Paired *t*-Test

6.23   The wattle thickness (in millimeters) of 15 randomly selected chickens was measured before and after treatment with PHA. Does treatment with PHA affect wattle thickness? (Data from F. McCorkle.)

Chicken Number	Pretreatment	Posttreatment
1	1.05	3.48
2	1.01	5.02
3	0.78	5.37
4	0.98	5.45
5	0.81	5.37
6	0.95	3.92
7	1.00	6.54
8	0.83	3.42
9	0.78	3.72
10	1.05	3.25
11	1.04	3.66
12	1.03	3.12
13	0.95	4.22
14	1.46	2.53
15	0.78	4.39

6.24 Data on resting and postexercise pulse rates were collected for 10 individuals between 19 and 22 years of age. We wish to know if there is a difference in preexercise and postexercise pulse rates.

Individual Number	Resting	Postexercise
1	108	136
2	60	90
3	70	78
4	54	108
5	54	102
6	72	92
7	101	118
8	96	176

6.25 For the situation in 6.24, the following data are for preexercise and postexercise body temperature. Is there a difference in the 2 body temperatures?

Individual Number	Resting	Postexercise
1	99.0	99.4
2	97.8	98.1
3	98.6	98.6
4	98.7	98.7
5	98.7	98.7
6	98.2	98.2
7	98.7	98.8
8	98.6	99.2

6.26 *Brucella abortus* antibody titers (pfc/10^6 cells) in 15 turkeys were measured before and after a period of stress. We wish to know if stress affects antibody titer.

Turkey Number	Before Stress	After Stress
1	20	17
2	18	14
3	19	16
4	18	19
5	17	14
6	14	18
7	17	8
8	10	10
9	13	12
10	16	15
11	20	8
12	17	6
13	16	17
14	19	5
15	8	3

6.27   Six laboratory mice were placed one at a time in a one-square-meter enclosure. The number of seconds in one minute that they were either near the wall or away from the wall was noted. We wish to know if mice spend more time by a wall than away from a wall (i.e., is there a "wall-seeking tendency" in this species?).

Mouse Number	Seconds by Wall	Seconds Away from Wall
1	50	10
2	35	25
3	28	32
4	45	15
5	31	29
6	55	5

The Wilcoxon Signed-Ranks Matched-Pairs Test

6.28   Ten individuals were asked to rate their feeling of well-being on a scale of 1 to 10 before and after taking an experimental drug. Does the drug change a person's sense of well-being?

Individual Number	Before Drug	After Drug
1	5	7
2	8	9
3	2	1
4	7	9
5	5	5
6	2	9
7	9	9
8	3	9
9	9	10
10	6	7

6.29   Assume that the variable in exercise 6.25 is not approximately normally distributed. Conduct a Wilcoxon test with these data.

6.30   Assume that the variable in exercise 6.26 is not approximately normally distributed. Conduct a Wilcoxon test with these data.

The Sign Test

6.31   Ten subjects were given an experimental drug and asked if their sense of well-being improved, became worse, or did not change after taking the drug. We wish to know if the drug is effective in improving one's sense of well-being. The results were as follows.

7 reported an improvement

2 reported no change

1 reported feeling worse

6.32   Conduct a sign test using the data in exercise 6.25.

6.33   Conduct a sign test using the data in exercise 6.26.

6.34   Conduct a sign test using the data in exercise 6.27.

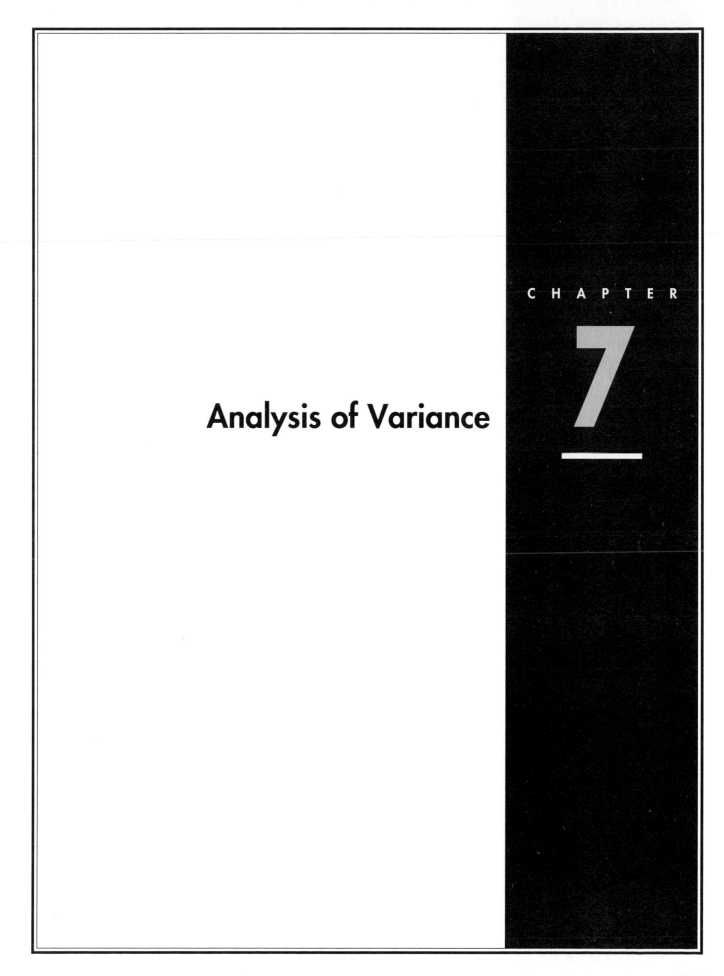

Analysis of Variance

Analysis of variance (ANOVA) is one of the most versatile and useful techniques of statistical inference. Analysis of variance is a complex subject, and we will touch here only on the basic concepts and the most common applications. Essentially, ANOVA is a technique of partitioning the variance in a set of data into several components in such a way that the contribution of each of these components to the overall data set may be assessed. The techniques of ANOVA are really most useful in situations where the researcher can carefully design and control experiments, but they may also be very useful for the analysis of several types of observational data under certain conditions.

Analysis of variance and proper experimental design are closely associated, and in fact, different techniques of ANOVA are specifically applicable to particular experimental designs. The 2 are not really separable. Before beginning an experiment utilizing ANOVA, one should carefully review the various experimental designs for which the various techniques of ANOVA are appropriate, as well as the assumptions of ANOVA.

THE RATIONALE OF ANOVA: AN ILLUSTRATION

The rationale of analyzing the variance of samples when our interest is in their means may be illustrated by this hypothetical example. Fifteen juniper pythons, all of similar age and size, were randomly assigned to one of 3 groups. Group A received a certain drug; group B received another drug; and group C, the control group, received a placebo. The heart rate of each snake was then determined to see if either or both of the drugs affects heart rate. The null hypothesis in an experiment such as this is that the means of all 3 populations are equal, or

$$H_0: \mu_A = \mu_B = \mu_C$$

Population, in this case, refers to all possible juniper pythons that might be given a particular treatment.

In a case like this, why could we not simply conduct a series of t-tests, comparing each group with each other group (i.e., group A with group B, A with C, and B with C)? Even if it were appropriate to do this, which it is not, it would not be very efficient. Making all possible comparisons of pairs among 10 treatments, for example, would require 45 t-tests! And why is it not appropriate to do this, regardless of the inefficiency involved? Suppose we set alpha at 0.05 for rejecting H_0 in any individual t-test (i.e., we will reject the null hypothesis that the means of any 2 groups are equal when $p \leq 0.05$). In such a situation there is a probability of 0.05 of making a type I error when comparing any 2 sample means. Thus, we would expect to make a type I error about one time in 20 t-tests. If we compared all possible group means for 10 groups (45 t-tests), we would expect a type I error to occur about twice, causing us to incorrectly reject the null hypothesis that all of the group means are equal. Analysis of variance is designed to overcome this problem.

Because all of the individual juniper pythons in the study were chosen from the same population or group, it may be assumed that all of the individuals (the "experimental units") involved in the experiment are more or less homogeneous. Any variation from one individual to another within a group is the normal variation we expect among individuals in a population; it is called **error variance (within-groups variance).** Because snakes from the available group of 15 were randomly assigned to the 3 treatment groups, we expect the error variance within each group to be approximately the same. Suppose we obtained the results shown in table 7.1.

Table 7.1 The Effect of Two Drugs on the Heart Rate of Juniper Pythons (Beats per Minute)

	Group A	Group B	Group C
	13	7	3
	15	6	5
	12	10	2
	14	9	4
	11	8	1
$\bar{x}$	13	8	3
s^2	2.50	2.50	2.50
		$s_t^2 = 19.124$	

Remember, the objective of ANOVA is to partition the variance in a set of data into various components and to determine the contribution of each of these components to the overall variation. First, we consider the overall variation in the complete data set (all 15 snakes considered together). This is called the total variance, and it is about 19.124 in this case. There are 2 sources of this variation. One source is the usual variation from one individual to another, caused by genetic and environmental differences among individuals, and it has nothing to do with the treatments the animals were given. This is called error variance. Note in table 7.1 that the variance in each group (the error variance) is the same (about 2.5). There is quite a difference between this error variance and the total variance, which tells us there is a source of variance that is not accounted for by the normal variance from one individual to another. Its source is the variance introduced by our treatments. The difference between the total variance in the data set and the error variance is called the **between-groups variance (treatment variance).**

The sampling distribution that describes the ratio of these 2 variances, or

$$\frac{\text{between-groups (treatment) variance}}{\text{error variance}}$$

is the *F* distribution. The *F* distribution is another theoretical probability distribution whose derivation need not concern us. It is based on 2 degrees of freedom, which, in ANOVA applications, are the between-groups (treatment) degrees of freedom (the number of treatments minus one) and the error degrees of freedom (the total number of observations in all groups minus the number of groups). A typical *F* distribution is shown in figure 7.1. The shaded portion of the curve is 0.05 of the total, and it is termed alpha, as before. The values of *F* that delimit this alpha region are found in table A.6, whose use will be described later.

When the treatments have no effect, virtually all of the variance in the data set will be due to error variance (which, you will recall, is the normal variance among individuals in a population), and the variance ratio will be very low.

If, at this point, you find yourself confused, that is as it should be. Confusion, they say, is the beginning of learning. Consider another imaginary outcome of this same imaginary experiment, shown in table 7.2. In this case the error variance and the total variance are practically the same, and we would probably conclude that most of the variation within the data set is attributable to the usual variation between individuals and that little or none of it results

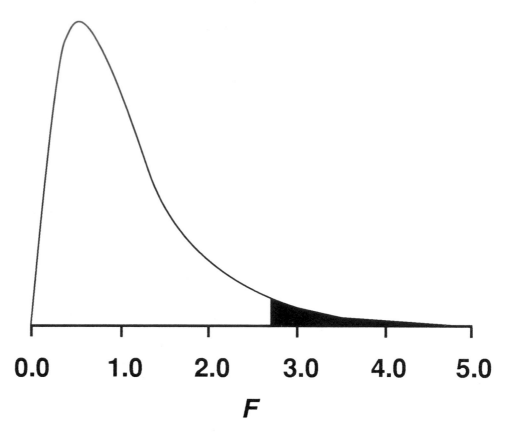

Figure 7.1
An F distribution.

from the treatments given. In this case we would no doubt accept H_0 and conclude that neither drug has an effect on heart rate. How we reach this decision is explained in the following sections.

Table 7.2   The Effect of Two Drugs on the Heart Rate of Juniper Pythons (Beats per Minute)

	Group A	Group B	Group C
	1	3	2
	3	5	1
	2	1	5
	5	4	4
	4	2	3
$\bar{x}$	3	3	3
s^2	2.50	2.50	2.50
		$s_t^2 = 2.14$	

THE ASSUMPTIONS OF ANOVA

There are several important assumptions of ANOVA, which should be adhered to rather closely. In particular the assumption that the error variances are equal should be tested anytime there is a suspicion that the error variances might not be equal. Example 7.4 is a situation in which one might wish to test this assumption. Later in this chapter we will see how this is done.

General Assumptions of ANOVA

1. Each of the groups is a random sample from the population of interest.
2. The measured variable is continuous (or if discrete, it may assume a large range of values).
3. Measurement is on a ratio or interval scale.
4. The error variances are equal.
5. The variable is approximately normally distributed.

Assumption 1 may not be violated! Randomization is usually achieved by randomly assigning the available experimental subjects to the various treatment groups, as in the juniper python illustration. When any of assumptions 2 through 5 are not met, one should consider one of the nonparametric methods discussed later in this chapter.

Several experimental designs are used with ANOVA, and each of these requires a somewhat different set of computations. Which design is chosen depends on the nature of the question being asked. In the following sections, we will examine some of the more common ANOVA designs.

THE COMPLETELY RANDOMIZED DESIGN ANOVA

Example 7.1 is an imaginary but fairly typical situation in which the completely randomized design ANOVA is useful. There are 3 sample means representing 3 treatments, one of which serves as the control. We wish to know if either or both of the treatments are significantly different from the control. These are random samples because the individual subjects (experimental units) were randomly assigned to the 3 groups.

EXAMPLE 7.1   An Experiment Utilizing the Completely Randomized Design

A group of 30 highly inbred mice, just weaned, were randomly divided into 3 groups of 10 mice each and were given 3 different diets. At the end of several weeks, the gain in weight of each mouse was determined. Group A (the control group) was fed regular laboratory mouse food; group B was fed potato chips, twinkies, and diet cola (the junk food diet); and group C was fed granola and organically grown prune juice (the health food diet). The results of the experiment are shown in table 7.3. We wish to determine if the mean weight gain among the 3 treatments (samples, groups) is significantly different. Suppose the results of our imaginary experiment were as follows.

Weight Gain in Mice		
Group A (Control)	Group B (Junk Food)	Group C (Health Food)
10.8	12.7	9.8
11.0	13.9	8.6
9.7	11.8	8.0
10.1	13.0	7.5
11.2	11.0	9.0
9.8	10.9	10.0
10.5	13.6	8.1
9.5	10.9	7.8
10.0	11.5	7.9
10.2	12.8	9.1

The null hypothesis is

$$H_0: \mu_A = \mu_B = \mu_C$$

and the alternative hypothesis is

$$H_1: \text{not all } \mu \text{ are equal.}$$

An experiment of this type is referred to as a **completely random design ANOVA with fixed effects (model I).** The design is called completely random because the experimental units (individual mice) are randomly assigned to the various treatment groups by the investigator. Since each experimental unit is from the same population, it is assumed that the variation among individuals within any treatment group is the variation usually expected among individuals in a population. Fixed effects (sometimes referred to as a model I ANOVA) means that the treatments to be used in the experiment are chosen by the investigator. This design may also be called a one-way ANOVA with fixed effects, since each observation (individual) in the data set is classified according to only one criterion—the group to which it is assigned.

Before beginning a discussion of how one proceeds to test the null hypothesis, we need to consider how and why this experiment was designed as it was. First, it is helpful in such an experiment if the error variance—the variance not associated with the treatments—can be kept to a minimum. This can often be accomplished by selecting experimental units (mice, in this case) that are as nearly alike as possible. For this experiment a group of inbred mice of the same age was used. Randomly assigning the experimental units to the treatment groups is crucial to ensure that variation among individuals that still exists (in spite of our best efforts to minimize it) is not associated with one group more than with any other, and that the variance within each group (the error variance) will be equal.

Once the sample has been properly selected and the experiment begins, it is necessary to ensure that all groups are treated identically, as far as possible, with respect to housing, water, temperature, and in every other way except for the factor being tested (diet, in this case). Only then may we feel confident that any difference in weight gain noted among the 3 groups is caused by diet and not by some other factor.

Testing the Null Hypothesis That All Treatment Means Are Equal

The first step in conducting an ANOVA is to test the null hypothesis that all of the treatment (group) means are equal, or

$$H_0: \mu_A = \mu_B = \ldots \mu_i$$

Recall that we expect the ratio of the between-groups variance to the error variance (the variance ratio, or F) to be approximately one when the null hypothesis is true, and that the sampling distribution that describes the variance ratio is the F distribution.

Example 7.1 illustrates the calculations for obtaining the variance ratio, F. The data of this experiment and the means of the 3 groups are given in table 7.3. The preliminary calculations needed to compute the variance ratio are given in table 7.4. We will go through these calculations step by step.

Table 7.3 Weight Gain by Mice Fed Mouse Food (Control—Group A), Junk Food (Group B), and Health Food (Group C) (Data from Example 7.1)

Group A	Group B	Group C
10.8	12.7	9.8
11.0	13.9	8.6
9.7	11.8	8.0
10.1	13.0	7.5
11.2	11.0	9.0
9.8	10.9	10.0
10.5	13.6	8.1
9.5	10.9	7.8
10.0	11.5	7.9
10.2	12.8	9.1
$\bar{x} = 10.28$	12.21	8.58
$n = 10$	10	10

1. Sum the observations for each group individually. These values are designated as Σx_A, Σx_B, and Σx_C. For the example, $\Sigma x_A = 102.8$, $\Sigma x_B = 122.1$, and $\Sigma x_C = 85.8$.

2. Divide the sum of the x values for each group by the number of observations in the group ($\frac{\Sigma x_i}{n_i}$). These are the means of the 3 groups and are designated as $\bar{x}_A$, $\bar{x}_B$, and $\bar{x}_C$. For the example,

$$\bar{x}_A = \frac{102.8}{10} = 10.28, \bar{x}_B = \frac{122.1}{10} = 12.21$$

and

$$\bar{x}_C = \frac{85.8}{10} = 8.58$$

3. For each group square the x values and sum them. These are designated as Σx^2_A, Σx^2_B, and Σx^2_C. (Some hand calculators with statistical functions store the sums of the squared values in a memory, and the sums may be recalled—consult your user's manual.) For the example, $\Sigma x^2_A = 1059.76$, $\Sigma x^2_B = 1502.41$, and $\Sigma x^2_C = 742.92$.

4. For each group, square the summed x values obtained in step 1. These values are designated as $(\Sigma x_A)^2$, $(\Sigma x_B)^2$, and $(\Sigma x_C)^2$. For the example, $(\Sigma x_A)^2 = (102.8)^2 = 10567.84$, $(\Sigma x_B)^2 = (122.1)^2 = 14908.41$, and $(\Sigma x_C)^2 = (85.8)^2 = 7361.64$.

5. Divide each of the values obtained in step 4 by its sample size and sum the results in the following manner:

$$\frac{(\Sigma x_A)^2}{n_A} + \frac{(\Sigma x_B)^2}{n_B} + \frac{(\Sigma x_C)^2}{n_C}$$

This value is designated as

$$\Sigma\left[\frac{(\Sigma x)^2}{n}\right]$$

For the example,

$$\Sigma\left[\frac{(\Sigma x)^2}{n}\right] = \left(\frac{10567.84}{10}\right) + \left(\frac{14908.41}{10}\right) + \left(\frac{7361.64}{10}\right) = 3283.78$$

The next few values to be calculated are for the overall sample and are shown in the right column of table 7.4.

6. Sum the values of n for each group. This is the total number of observations and is designated as n_t. For the example, $n_t = 10 + 10 + 10 = 30$.

7. Sum the sums of the x values for each group. This value is designated as Σx_t. For the example, $\Sigma x_t = 102.8 + 122.1 + 85.8 = 310.7$.

8. Sum the sums of the x^2 values for each group. This value is designated as Σx^2_t. For the example, $\Sigma x^2_t = 1059.76 + 1502.41 + 742.92 = 3305.09$.

9. Square the value for Σx_t that was found in step 7. Caution: this is not obtained by adding the $(\Sigma x)^2$ values of the groups. For the example, $(\Sigma x_t)^2 = 310.7^2 = 96534.49$.

10. Divide $(\Sigma x_t)^2$ from step 9 by n_t. This value is designated as $\frac{(\Sigma x_t)^2}{n_t}$. For the example,

$$\frac{(\Sigma x_t)^2}{n_t} = \frac{96534.49}{30} = 3217.82$$

Recall that earlier we mentioned an important value called the sum of squares (refer to chapter 3), which, when divided by a number we referred to as $n - 1$, or degrees of freedom, yields an estimate of variance, also called a mean square. We now calculate 3 sums of squares using the calculations we have just done.

Table 7.4   Preliminary ANOVA Calculations for the Data from Table 7.3

Value	Group A	Group B	Group C	Total
n	10	10	10	$n_t = 30$
$\overline{x}$	10.28	12.21	8.58	
Σx	102.8	122.1	85.8	$x_t = 310.7$
Σx^2	1059.76	1502.41	742.92	$x^2_t = 3305.09$
$(\Sigma x)^2$	10567.84	14908.41	7361.64	$(\Sigma x_t)^2 = 96534.49$
$\dfrac{(\Sigma x)^2}{n}$	1056.84	1490.84	736.16	$\dfrac{(\Sigma x_t)^2}{n_t} = 3217.82$
		$\Sigma\left[\dfrac{(\Sigma x)^2}{n}\right] = 3283.84$		

The total sum of squares, SS_t, is given by

$$SS_t = \Sigma x^2_t - \frac{(\Sigma x_t)^2}{n_t} \tag{7.1}$$

The between-groups (treatment) sum of squares, SS_b, is given by

$$SS_b = \Sigma \left[\frac{(\Sigma x)^2}{n} \right] - \frac{(\Sigma x_t)^2}{n_t} \tag{7.2}$$

3283.78 − 3217.82 *(handwritten)*

and the error (within-groups) sum of squares, SS_e, is given by

$$SS_e = SS_t - SS_b \tag{7.3}$$

To convert these sums of squares into mean squares, we must divide each by an appropriate degrees of freedom. The between-groups degrees of freedom (df_b) is the number of groups minus 1 ($k - 1$). The total degrees of freedom (df_t) is $n_t - 1$, and the error degrees of freedom (df_e) is obtained by subtracting the between-groups degrees of freedom from the total degrees of freedom. We usually arrange the sums of squares, degrees of freedom, and mean squares in a tabular form like tables 7.5 and 7.6. The mean squares of interest are obtained by dividing the sums of squares by their appropriate degrees of freedom. F (the variance ratio) is obtained by dividing the between-groups mean square by the error mean square.

Table 7.5   Generalized ANOVA Table

Source of Variation	SS	df	Mean Square (MS)	F
Between-Groups	SS_b	df_b	$\dfrac{SS_b}{df_b}$	$\dfrac{MS_b}{MS_e}$
Error	SS_e	df_e	$\dfrac{SS_e}{df_e}$	
Total	SS_t	df_t		

Table 7.6   ANOVA Table for Mouse Diet Example

Source of Variation	SS	df	Mean Square (MS)	F
Between-Groups	65.96	2	32.98	41.81
Error	21.31	27	0.789	
Total	87.27	29		

Work through the example to ensure comprehension! We now consult table A.6, "Critical Values of the F Distribution," to see if we may reject H_0. The top row of the table gives degrees of freedom for the numerator mean square (the between-groups mean square), and the left column gives degrees of freedom for the denominator mean square (the error mean square). In this case the degrees of freedom are 2 and 27. If our calculated value of F is equal to or greater than the tabular value of F, we may reject H_0. The table value for 2 and 27 degrees of freedom (2 and 25, since 2 and 27 is not tabulated) is 3.39. Since our calculated value is much greater than this, we may reject H_0 and conclude that the means of the 3 treatments are not all equal, $p < 0.05$ (i.e., that one or more of the treatment means differs from the others).

Multiple Comparisons

Which means are different from which other means? At this point we cannot say. There are a number of different techniques for testing the differences between individual means in an ANOVA (called **multiple comparisons**). The specific technique depends to some extent on whether the investigator planned to compare certain groups of means or individual means with certain other means before the experiment was conducted. These are called planned comparisons. In other cases the investigator does not know before the experiment is conducted which means are to be compared to which other means, and in fact, may wish to compare all possible pairs of means with each other. These are called unplanned comparisons. Whereas the techniques designed specifically for planned comparisons are usually not applicable to unplanned comparisons, those techniques designed for unplanned comparisons may be used in the case of planned comparisons. In this chapter we will deal with only one technique for unplanned comparisons, the extended Tukey test for multiple comparisons, because it is computationally relatively simple. There are a number of such tests that one may use.

In example 7.1 we rejected H_0: $\mu_A = \mu_B = \mu_C$. The error mean square for this test was 0.789 with 27 df, and n for all 3 treatments was 10. We may now compute a critical value that the difference between any 2 means must equal or exceed to be considered significantly different from each other. This critical value (CV) for samples of equal size is given by

$$CV = q \sqrt{\frac{MS_e}{n}} \tag{7.4}$$

where MS_e is the error mean square, n is the sample size, and q is the studentized range value, found in table A.7, "Critical Values of q for the Tukey Test."

When the sizes of the 2 samples being compared are unequal, the CV is given by

$$CV = q \sqrt{\frac{MS_e}{n_{1,2}}} \tag{7.5}$$

where $n_{1,2}$ is the geometric mean of the 2 sample sizes and is calculated by

$$n_{1,2} = \frac{2n_1 n_2}{n_1 + n_2} \tag{7.6}$$

The value for q is found in table A.7. The top row of the table gives the number of groups (treatments), designated by k, and the left column gives the error degrees of freedom. The cell entry is the value of q. Thus, the critical value is

$$CV = 3.53 \sqrt{\frac{0.789}{10}} = 0.9915$$

Since there is no entry in the table for 27 df, we use the next lower df, which is 24. Any error caused by doing this is a conservative one. If a more accurate value for q is needed, it may be obtained by interpolation. We now calculate the absolute difference between each pair of means.

$$A - B = 10.28 - 12.21 = 1.93$$
$$A - C = 10.28 - 8.58 = 1.70$$
$$B - C = 12.25 - 8.58 = 3.67$$

Since the differences between the various pairs of means are all larger than the CV, we may conclude that all of the means are significantly different from each other at the 0.05 level of significance. A diet of potato chips, twinkies, and diet cola induces a greater rate of weight gain in laboratory mice than does regular mouse food, which in turn induces more weight gain than does granola and organically grown prune juice.

An alternative way of considering this same information when sample sizes are all equal is to compute confidence intervals of the group means, which are simply

$$\bar{x} \pm \frac{CV}{2}$$

(Note that this is not the way one computes a confidence interval for a single mean, as in chapter 5.) For the example, these 95% confidence intervals are $\frac{\bar{x} \pm 0.9915}{2}$ and are shown below.

Treatment	Mean	95% CI
A	10.28	9.78 to 10.77
B	12.21	11.71 to 12.71
C	8.58	8.08 to 9.08

Means whose confidence intervals do not overlap are considered to be significantly different at the indicated level of significance. In this case, since we used 95% confidence intervals, we conclude that all 3 treatment means are significantly different at the 95% level. This information may also be presented graphically, as shown in figure 7.2. The vertical lines represent confidence intervals. Again, means whose confidence intervals do not overlap are considered to be significantly different.

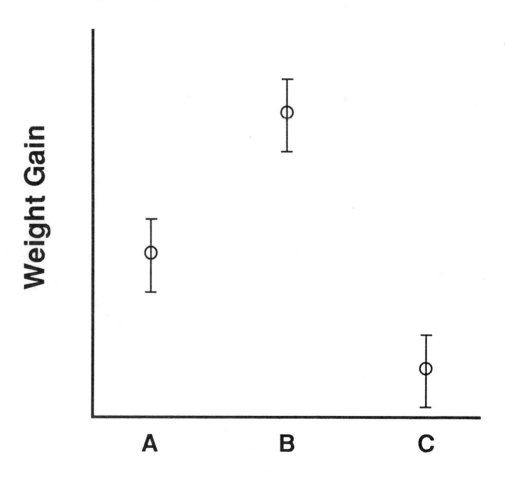

Figure 7.2
The 95% confidence interval for the means of example 7.1.

The Completely Randomized Design with Fixed Effects Using Observational Data

"Treatments" in ANOVA are not necessarily something that an experimenter "does" to groups of individuals, as in example 7.1. Rather, they may be some factor that differs from population to population if we feel relatively confident that the populations are similar except with respect to this factor (this is not always a valid assumption). The following example may help to clarify this.

EXAMPLE 7.2 A Completely Randomized Design Using Observational Data

Random samples of 20 sticklebacks (a small minnow) were collected from 3 small lakes and 3 small streams in a given area. We wish to know if these populations differ in total length (in millimeters) among these 6 habitats. The data are shown in table 7.7. ■

Table 7.7 Data for Example 7.2

Lake A	Lake B	Lake C	Stream A	Stream B	Stream C
31	36	28	47	47	38
32	30	38	48	37	36
34	32	31	50	41	48
34	37	32	42	38	43
35	35	29	44	32	42
30	32	38	34	45	31
33	32	40	41	42	40
32	37	36	40	40	45
37	39	43	44	43	42
33	28	34	47	40	49
36	32	32	39	39	39
30	31	39	47	45	30
32	35	31	43	41	42
39	40	36	40	39	39
30	36	28	38	32	38
29	31	39	32	48	35
42	32	32	41	32	49
39	27	38	45	45	40
37	35	29	42	41	43
29	31	32	37	38	42

This is a fixed-effects model, since the habitats (treatments) were not chosen at random but were selected by the investigator. The term "treatment" in this situation does not have its usual meaning, since nothing was treated. Rather, treatment refers here to the locations from which the fish were sampled. Note that in this situation the investigator did not manipulate the situation beyond choosing the habitats to be sampled. Thus, the data are **observational data** rather than **experimental data.**

The calculations for a completely randomized design using observational data are exactly the same as when using experimental data. The major difference is in the interpretation. In example 7.1 we can be fairly certain that different diets caused differences in weight gain in our experimental animals because each animal was randomly assigned to each treatment group. In situations like example 7.2, it would not be accurate to conclude that different lakes or streams cause differences in the size of sticklebacks (if such differences are revealed by the ANOVA) because individual fish were not randomly assigned to the various habitats: they were already there. Thus, while we may detect differences among habitats, we should not conclude that the habitats directly cause the differences in the same sense that the diets in example 7.1 could be considered to be the cause of the differences in weight gain.

If you worked your way through example 7.1 and tried your hand at a couple of the problems at the end of this chapter, you have developed a feeling about ANOVA by calculator, pencil, and paper, and if you are more or less normal, that feeling is probably somewhat negative. Accordingly, the computer solution to example 7.2 is given in figure 7.5 at the end of this chapter.

The Completely Randomized Design with Random Effects

In examples 7.1 and 7.2 we were dealing with fixed-effects models (sometimes called model I ANOVA) because the treatments (diets, habitats) were selected by the investigator and we had no interest in generalizing the results to other diets or other habitats. In other words the questions asked were "Do these three diets differ with respect to weight gain induced in mice?" and "Is there a difference in the size of sticklebacks among these 3 lakes and 3 streams?"

On occasion we wish to ask a somewhat different question, such as "Is diet an important factor in weight gain?" In such a case, we might select a number of different diets *at random* from a large population of different possible diets and test these much as we did earlier. In this case, however, the treatments (diets) are not selected by the investigator but rather are chosen at random from a *population* of possible diets (thus, random effects). An ANOVA design using random effects is sometimes called a **random-effects (model II) ANOVA.** In this case the null hypothesis is that not all diets are equal, and the alternative hypothesis is that one or more of the diets are different from the others.

We do not conduct a multiple-comparisons test in this type of ANOVA if the null hypothesis is rejected, since we have no interest in which diets are different from which others. Why is this? If the experiment were repeated, it is highly likely that different treatments (which, as you recall, were selected at random) would be used. Our question was "Does diet affect weight gain in mice?" If the overall ANOVA, which is conducted the same for the random-effects model as for the fixed-effects model, is significant, then the answer is yes.

EXAMPLE 7.3   A Completely Randomized Design
with Random Effects

A fisheries biologist wished to determine if the fecundity of a particular species of fish might be influenced by habitat (i.e., if different lakes differed with respect to the fecundity of this species).   ■

To answer this question, the biologist might randomly select a number of lakes from a larger population of lakes and conduct a one-way ANOVA using the completely random design with random effects. The ANOVA is conducted exactly as in the previous examples, except that multiple comparisons are not conducted. If the null hypothesis is rejected, the conclusion is that habitat affects fecundity. How it might differ from one particular lake to another is not a question in the random-effects model, since if another random sample had been chosen, it would very likely include different lakes.

THE RANDOMIZED COMPLETE BLOCKS DESIGN

Suppose that in example 7.1 our interest was in a wild population of white-footed deer mice rather than in highly inbred laboratory mice. We might expect that genetic variability would be fairly high in such a population. Using the completely random design discussed above, this additional variance due to genetic differences and age differences among the experimental units would be unrecognizable as such and would, in fact, be a part of the error variance. This larger error variance would have the effect of reducing the variance ratio and making it more difficult to reject the null hypothesis.

The **randomized complete blocks design** provides a way to deal with this problem. In this design individuals are "blocked" (grouped) according to the characteristic whose variance we wish to identify and "partition out." In this case we would group individuals according to litters, since it is likely that members of the same litter are genetically similar and of the same age. Note that each individual observation (each mouse) is classified according to 2 criteria (diet and litter) and that only one individual occupies each possible combination of diet and litter. Thus, this particular design is sometimes called a two-way ANOVA without replication. It is a fixed-effects model (model I), since treatments to be given were chosen by the investigator.

As in the completely randomized design, the null hypothesis in a randomized complete blocks design is that the treatment means are equal. If the null hypothesis is rejected, we may then conduct a multiple comparisons test as described previously to test which means might be different from which other means.

EXAMPLE 7.4   A Randomized Complete Blocks Design

Ten litters of white-footed deer mice of approximately the same age were selected. One member of each litter was randomly assigned to 1 of the 3 treatment groups (the diets of example 7.1), and their weight gain was determined as before. The results are given in table 7.8.   ■

Table 7.8   Weight Gain by White-footed Deer Mice Fed Mouse Food, Junk Food, and Health Food

	Litter Number	Treatments Group A	Group B	Group C	Σx_r	$(\Sigma x_r)^2$
	1	11.8	13.6	9.2	34.6	1197.16
	2	12.0	14.4	9.6	36.0	1296.00
	3	10.7	12.8	8.6	32.1	1030.41
	4	9.1	13.0	8.5	30.6	936.36
Blocks	5	12.1	13.4	9.8	35.3	1246.09
	6	9.8	10.9	10.0	30.7	942.49
	7	10.5	13.6	9.2	33.3	1108.89
	8	10.5	11.9	8.8	31.2	973.44
	9	9.0	10.5	6.9	26.4	696.96
	10	11.2	13.8	10.1	35.1	1232.01
	$\bar{x}$	10.67	12.79	9.07		
	Σx_c	106.7	127.9	90.7	$\Sigma x_t = 325.30$	
	$(\Sigma x_c)^2$	11384.89	16358.41	8226.49		

Several features about this design require attention. Treatments, in this case, are the different diets and represent the factor in which we have an interest. Blocks, which are the individual litters, represent the source of variation we regard as extraneous and we wish to remove (or partition out) from what would otherwise be a part of the error variance. Each treatment contains one and only one member of each block. In the example we would randomly select one member of each litter for each treatment. The total number of observations in such a design is therefore the number of treatments (diets) $\times$ the number of blocks (litters).

The calculations for the randomized complete blocks design are similar to those for the completely randomized design except that they are a bit more extensive because the objective is to partition the variance into more components. In this case we desire to partition the total sum of squares into a sum of squares associated with the treatments, a sum of squares associated with the blocks, and an error sum of squares. The results of the preliminary calculations (up to step 5) for our example are shown in table 7.8.

1. Sum each row. These values are designated as Σx_r.
2. Sum each column. These values are designated as Σx_c.
3. Sum either the column totals or the row totals from step 1 or 2 (the result should be the same either way). This is designated as Σx_t. It is the value in the lower right of table 7.8.
4. Square the sums of the rows from step 1. These values are designated as $(\Sigma x_r)^2$. Sum the squared sums and divide this by the number of treatments (columns). This value is designated as

$$\frac{\Sigma(\Sigma x_r)^2}{c}$$

where c is the number of columns (treatments). For the example, this value is

$$\frac{1197.16 + 1296.0 + \ldots 1232.01}{3} = 3553.27$$

5. Square the sums of the columns from step 2. These values are designated as $(\Sigma x_c)^2$. Sum the squared sums of the columns and divide this value by the number of rows (blocks). This value is designated as

$$\frac{\Sigma(\Sigma x_c)^2}{r}$$

For the example, this value is

$$\frac{11384.89 + 16358.41 + 8226.49}{10} = \frac{35969.79}{10} = 3596.98$$

6. Square all of the observations in all of the treatments and sum the squares. This value is designated as

$$\Sigma x^2{}_t$$

For the example, this value is

$$(11.8)^2 + (12)^2 + \ldots (10.1)^2 = 3631.47$$

7. Square the grand total and divide by the total number of observations. This value is designated as

$$\frac{(\Sigma x_t)^2}{n_t}$$

For the example, this value is

$$\frac{(325.30)^2}{30} = 3527.336$$

This completes the preliminary calculations. The steps involved in computing the sums of squares and degrees of freedom required to complete the ANOVA are given below, and the values for the example are given in the ANOVA table (table 7.9).

1. Total sum of squares.

$$SS_t = \Sigma x_t^2 - \frac{(\Sigma x_t)^2}{n_t} \qquad (7.7)$$

For the example, this value is

$$3631.47 - 3527.336 = 104.134$$

2. The sum of squares for treatments (columns) is

$$SS_c = \frac{\Sigma(\Sigma x_c)^2}{r} - \frac{(\Sigma x_t)^2}{n_t} \qquad (7.8)$$

where r is the number of rows (blocks). For the example, this value is

$$\frac{35969.79}{10} - 3527.336 = 69.643$$

3. The sum of squares for blocks (rows) is

$$SS_r = \frac{\Sigma(\Sigma x_r)^2}{c} - \frac{(\Sigma x_t)^2}{n_t} \quad\quad (7.9)$$

where c is the number of columns (treatments). For the example, this is

$$\frac{10659.811}{3} - 3527.336 = 25.934$$

4. The error sum of squares is

$$SS_e = SS_t - SS_c - SS_r \quad\quad (7.10)$$

For the example, this value is

$$104.134 - 69.643 - 25.934 = 8.557$$

The degrees of freedom for these sums of squares are

Total degrees of freedom, $df_t = n_t - 1$. For the example, this is $30 - 1 = 29$.

Column (treatment) degrees of freedom, $df_c = \text{columns} - 1$. For the example, this is $3 - 1 = 2$.

Row (block) degrees of freedom, $df_r = \text{rows} - 1$. For the example, this is $10 - 1 = 9$.

Error degrees of freedom, $df_e = df_t - df_c - df_r$. For the example, this is $29 - 2 - 9 = 18$.

Table 7.9 is the ANOVA table for the example. The variance ratio, F, for treatments is found by dividing the treatment mean square by the error mean square. The critical value of F is found in table A.6 for 2 and 20 degrees of freedom (18 is not tabulated). For the example, the critical value is 3.49 for alpha $= 0.05$. Since our calculated F value is much larger than this, we reject H_0 and conclude that diet has a significant effect on weight gain in white-footed deer mice. It is also possible to test for significant differences among blocks, but this is usually of little or no interest. In the example, we really have no interest in knowing if there are differences among individual litters with respect to weight gain on the various diets. The blocks, as you will recall, were used to partition out this effect from the error variance and thereby reduce it.

Table 7.9 ANOVA Table for Example 7.4

Source	SS	df	Mean Square	F
Columns (Diets, Treatments)	69.643	2	34.82	73.31
Rows (Litters, Blocks)	25.934	9	2.88	
Error	8.557	18	0.475	
Total	104.134	29		

A very common use of the randomized complete blocks design is when one desires to make 3 or more repeated measurements on the same individual. Thus, it may be used in much the same way that the paired t-test is used, except that more than 2 measurements are involved. (The paired t-test is, in fact, a special case of the randomized complete blocks design.) When used in this way, the randomized complete blocks design is sometimes called "repeated measures ANOVA."

EXAMPLE 7.5 A Randomized Complete Blocks Design Using Repeated Measures

The convict cichlid is one of several fish species that exhibits biparental care of eggs and fry. An experiment was conducted to determine if male convict cichlids might spend more time in direct offspring care with fry than with eggs. Accordingly, the time eight males spent in this activity (in seconds) during a 15 minute observation period was determined for 5 consecutive days. The eggs hatched after 2 days and for several days after that the fry were attached to the substrate by sticky "pads" on their heads. The results are given in table 7.10.

Table 7.10 Brooding Time (sec/15 min) by Male Convict Cichlids

Male Number	Day 1	Day 2	Day 3	Day 4	Day 5
1	11.9	2.2	57.9	259.5	200.4
2	42.7	60.7	71.2	163.3	228.1
3	15.8	14.8	311.3	283.9	436.3
4	191.2	148.8	437.8	319.2	462.6
5	3.5	187.3	281.4	410.4	373.7
6	23.7	0.0	98.6	185.7	106.8
7	0.0	0.0	102.4	400.7	386.9
8	33.5	107.5	193.5	317.8	337.3

Data from D. Dickens ■

In this case days are treatments, and individual males are blocks. The randomized complete blocks design is appropriate in this case because we wish to repeatedly measure the same males, and we wish to partition out the individual variation among males. You will note that this is considerable in this example and might well be large enough to mask any treatment effect if it were a part of the error variance. The calculations for this example are exactly the same as for the preceding example. The computer solution for this example is given in figure 7.6. The results lead us to conclude that we may reject the null hypotheses that the treatment means are equal, and that days 1 and 2 were not significantly different from each other but were significantly lower than days 3, 4, and 5. We conclude that males spend less time brooding eggs than brooding fry.

CAUTION

In a randomized complete blocks ANOVA, an important assumption is that interaction between the treatments and blocks is absent. Interaction means that treatments might affect individuals in one block differently than individuals in another block, or that the combined effect of the treatment and block factors somehow produce a result that is greater than the sum of their individual effects. If interaction is suspected, the factorial design, discussed in the following section, is appropriate.

THE FACTORIAL DESIGN

In many situations 2 or more factors (treatments) interact with each other to produce effects beyond the sum of the effects of the 2 acting alone. In other words, factors (treatments) may interact either synergistically or antagonistically. For example, there are a number of medications that should not be taken together. Either drug taken alone might produce its desired effect, but when taken together they interact in some harmful way.

When **interaction** among 2 or more factors is suspected, the **factorial design** is appropriate. Note that it is similar to the randomized complete blocks design, except that the blocks as well as the treatments both represent factors in which we have an interest and that each block × treatment cell consists of replicated observations. You will recall that in the randomized complete blocks design, each block × treatment cell contained only one observation. In the factorial design, we usually speak of blocks (rows) as one major treatment effect and of treatments (columns) as the other major treatment effect in which we have an interest. Since each individual is classified according to 2 criteria—the 2 main treatments—and since there are several individuals (replicates) within each combination of the 2 treatments, this design is sometimes called two-way ANOVA with replication.

EXAMPLE 7.6   A Factorial Design ANOVA

Consider another mouse diet experiment similar to the 2 used to illustrate the completely randomized and the randomized complete blocks designs. In this experiment, however, we wish to determine the effect of diet, the effect of stress, and the interaction of these 2 factors, if any, on weight gain. We could conduct 2 separate experiments—onc on diet and one on stress—but this would give us no information on their possible interaction.

For this excperiment we select 32 highly inbred mice of the same age and sex (to minimize the error variance) and assign them at random to 4 groups. One group will receive the potato chip-twinkie-cola diet (junk food diet = J) and will listen to rap music eight hours each day (high stress = H). This group will be designated as JH. Another group will have the same diet but will listen to elevator music for eight hours each day (low stress = L). We will designate this group JL. A third group will receive regular mouse food (R) and will listen to rap music (H). We will designate this group RH. The fourth group will receive the regular diet (R) and will listen to elevator music (L). This is the RL group. All 4 groups will be housed under identical conditions. Thus, the 2 variables under study are arranged in all 4 possible combinations.   ■

It is convenient to arrange the data and the preliminary calculations as shown in table 7.11. We have an interest in 2 main effects (or treatments), diet and stress, and a possible interaction effect, which we wish to detect if it is present. We test 3 null hypotheses in a situation like this: $H_{0_1}: \mu_L = \mu_H$, $H_{0_2}: \mu_R = \mu_J$, and H_{0_3}: Interaction = 0. The row margins give the means and sums for diets, one of the major effects; and the column margins give the means and sums for stress, the other main effect. We proceed with the ANOVA as follows (see table 7.11).

Table 7.11 Data and Preliminary ANOVA Calculations for the Mouse Diet—Stress Interaction Example (Weight Gain, in Milligrams, in One Week)

	Low Stress	High Stress	
J Diet	132 $\bar{x}_{LJ} = 132.5$ 128 142 $\Sigma x_{LJ} = 1060$ 131 135 $n_{LJ} = 8$ 120 139 133	157 $\bar{x}_{HJ} = 152.3$ 143 162 $\Sigma x_{HJ} = 1218$ 150 149 $n_{HJ} = 8$ 140 159 158	$\bar{x}_J = 142.4$ $\Sigma x_J = 2278$ $n_J = 16$
R Diet	120 $\bar{x}_{LR} = 124.8$ 131 122 $\Sigma x_{LR} = 998$ 129 120 $n_{LR} = 8$ 119 134 123	130 $\bar{x}_{RH} = 132.0$ 142 131 $\Sigma x_{RH} = 1056$ 124 124 $n_{RH} = 8$ 131 143 131	$\bar{x}_R = 128.38$ $\Sigma x_R = 2054$ $n_R = 16$
	$\bar{x}_L = 128.7$	$\bar{x}_H = 142.13$	$\Sigma x_t = 4332$
	$\Sigma x_L = 2058$	$\Sigma x_H = 2274$	$\Sigma x_t^2 = 591{,}136$
	$n_L = 16$	$n_H = 16$	$n_t = 32$

1. The total sum of squares is given by

$$SS_t = \Sigma x_t^2 - \frac{(\Sigma x_t)^2}{n_t} \tag{7.11}$$

which, for the example, is

$$591136 - \frac{(4332)^2}{32} = 4691.5$$

2. The sum of squares for stress is

$$SS_s = \frac{(\Sigma x_L)^2}{n_L} + \frac{(\Sigma x_H)^2}{n_H} - \frac{(\Sigma x_t)^2}{n_t} \tag{7.12}$$

For the example, this is

$$\frac{(2058)^2}{16} + \frac{(2274)^2}{16} - \frac{(4332)^2}{32} = 1458$$

3. The sum of squares for diet is

$$SS_d = \frac{(\Sigma x_J)^2}{n_J} + \frac{(\Sigma x_R)^2}{n_R} - \frac{(\Sigma x_t)^2}{n_t} \tag{7.13}$$

For the example, this is

$$\frac{(2278)^2}{16} + \frac{(2054)^2}{16} - \frac{(4332)^2}{32} = 1568$$

4. The sum of squares for interaction is

$$SS_i = \frac{(\Sigma x_{HR})^2}{n_{HR}} + \frac{(\Sigma x_{LR})^2}{n_{LR}} + \frac{(\Sigma x_{HJ})^2}{n_{HJ}} + \frac{(\Sigma x_{IJ})^2}{n_{IJ}} - \frac{(\Sigma x_t)^2}{n_t} - SS_s - SS_d \quad \textbf{(7.14)}$$

For the example, this value is

$$\frac{(1060)^2}{8} + \frac{(998)^2}{8} + \frac{(1218)^2}{8} + \frac{(1056)^2}{8}$$
$$- \frac{(4332)^2}{32} - 1458 - 1568 = 312.5$$

5. The error sum of squares is

$$SS_e = SS_t - (SS_s + SS_d + SS_i) \quad \textbf{(7.15)}$$

For the example, this is

$$4561 - (1458 + 1568 + 312.5) = 1222.5$$

The degrees of freedom for each main effect is

$$\text{groups} - 1$$

For the example, in both cases this is

$$2 - 1 = 1$$

The degrees of freedom or interaction is

$$\text{df for one main effect} \times \text{df for the other main effect}$$

For the example, this is

$$1 \times 1 = 1$$

The total degrees of freedom is

$$n_t - 1$$

which, for the example, is

$$32 - 1 = 31$$

and the error degrees of freedom is

$$df_e = df_t - df_s - df_d - df_i$$

which, for the example, is

$$31 - 1 - 1 - 1 = 28$$

The sums of squares, degrees of freedom, and variances are arranged in an ANOVA table, as shown in table 7.12.

Table 7.12 ANOVA Table for the Data from Table 7.11

Source	df	SS	Mean Square
Stress	1	1458	1458
Diet	1	1568	1568
Interaction	1	312.5	312.5
Error	28	1353	48.32
Total	31	4691.5	

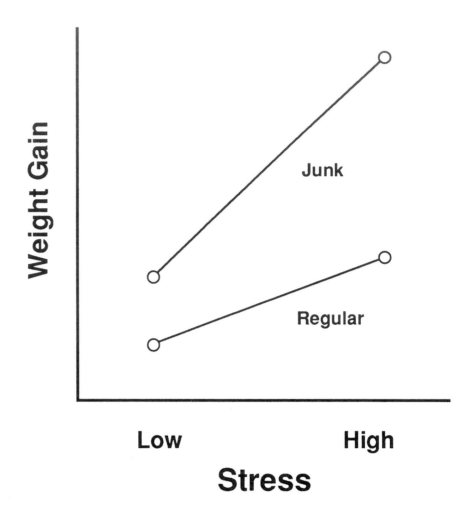

Figure 7.3
Graphic representation of the
cell means for example 7.6.

We now compute 3 *F* ratios: one for stress, one for diet, and one for interaction. Using the appropriate degrees of freedom, we consult table A.6. If our calculated value of *F* equals or exceeds the tabular value of *F*, we reject the appropriate null hypothesis. For the example,

$$F_{(stress)} = \frac{MS_s}{MS_e} = \frac{1458}{48.32} = 30.18 \text{ with } 1,28 \text{ df}$$

$$F_{(diet)} = \frac{MS_d}{MS_e} = \frac{1568}{48.32} = 32.46 \text{ with } 1,28 \text{ df}$$

$$F_{(int)} = \frac{MS_i}{MS_e} = \frac{312.5}{48.32} = 6.47 \text{ with } 1,28 \text{ df}$$

We compare these calculated *F* ratios with the tabular value of *F* for 1 and 30 df (since 28 is not tabulated), and we find that we may reject H_{0_1} and conclude that there is a significant effect of stress. We may also reject H_{0_2} and conclude that there is a significant effect of diet. Finally, we may reject H_{0_3} and conclude that there is a significant interaction of diet and stress. The highest weight gain was induced in individuals exposed to the junk food diet and high stress, and the lowest weight gain was induced in individuals exposed to the regular diet and low stress. Results of this nature are sometimes easier to interpret graphically, as shown in figure 7.3. No interaction is indicated when the lines drawn between the means are parallel.

The factorial design is not restricted to 2 levels of each treatment, as in the preceding example, but may include as many levels of the treatments as desired by the investigator. Example 7.7 illustrates a factorial design using 2 levels of one main effect and 3 levels of a second main effect. We will not go through the calculations for this example since they are the same regardless of the number of levels of each main effect.

EXAMPLE 7.7 A Factorial Design with More Than Two Levels of One of the Main Effects

An evolutionary biologist selected samples of road warblers (museum specimens) of both sexes from 3 locations: Eastern North America, Western North America, and the Intermountain region of North America. Ten individuals who were classified by these 2 criteria (sex and location) were selected at random, and their culmen (bill) lengths were measured. The results were as follows.

	Location		
	Eastern	Western	Intermountain
Females	50.1	53.4	54.0
	52.8	55.2	49.1
	50.8	51.0	60.5
	58.8	59.3	57.8
	59.7	61.5	48.7
	49.0	61.2	57.0
	58.8	57.8	61.1
	62.2	50.1	62.8
	57.8	56.0	59.8
	61.2	56.5	60.3
Males	46.5	57.5	49.1
	44.4	59.3	51.8
	42.0	62.4	55.3
	51.1	61.1	43.6
	45.8	59.9	50.1
	46.3	55.6	51.0
	41.8	56.8	49.0
	52.0	59.2	48.8
	46.5	50.4	52.0
	39.0	47.8	43.0

The computer solution to this problem is given in figure 7.7 at the end of this chapter.

TESTING THE ASSUMPTION OF EQUALITY OF WITHIN-GROUPS VARIANCES

As we have previously seen, one of the more important assumptions for any ANOVA is that the error variances are equal. This is often the case, since they presumably represent a common population variance. When individuals from a population are randomly assigned to treatments in a carefully controlled experiment, and assuming that the treatments do not in some way affect variability of a measured response, homogeneity of within-groups variance usually results. In example 7.1, which is a fairly typical application of a completely randomized design, the use of genetically similar individuals randomized among treatment groups should result in homogeneity of error variances. A design like example 7.4 is also expected to produce homogeneous variances because of blocking. Consider example 7.2, concerning the length of sticklebacks from six different habitats. In this case individuals could not be randomly assigned to the different habitats, since they were already there, and it would be unwise to assume that the variances among these 6 populations are equal.

The method of testing for the equality of error variances that we will use is called Bartlett's chi-square test for the homogeneity of variances. This test should only be used when the variable is reasonably normally distributed. The null hypothesis for this test is that the population variances of the various groups are equal. We will use example 7.2, reproduced as a table in example 7.8, to illustrate this test.

EXAMPLE 7.8   Group Means and Variances from Example 7.2

	$\overline{x}$	s^2	$ln\ s_i^2$
Lake A	33.70	13.484	2.602
Lake B	33.40	12.147	2.497
Lake C	34.25	19.882	2.990
Stream A	42.05	21.945	3.089
Stream B	40.25	21.776	3.080
Stream C	40.55	26.892	3.292

The equation

$$\chi^2 = [\Sigma(n_i - 1)]ln\ s_w^2 - \Sigma(n_i - 1)ln\ s_i^2 \tag{7.16}$$

has a chi-square distribution.

The chi-square (χ^2) distribution is yet another sampling distribution based on a theoretical probability distribution. It describes the distribution of variances of repeated samples, and its derivation need not concern us. Figure 7.4 is a chi-square distribution with 5 degrees of freedom. Table A.3 gives the critical values of chi-square that delimit the indicated proportions of the distribution at various degrees of freedom.

Bartlett's chi-square is computed in the following manner.

1. Convert the variances of the groups into their natural logarithms. These values, given in example 7.8, are designated as $ln\ s_i^2$.
2. Sum the degrees of freedom for the groups. This value is designated as $\Sigma(n_i - 1)$. For the example, this is

$$19 + 19 + 19 + 19 + 19 + 19 = 114$$

3. For each group multiply the degrees of freedom of the group by the variance of the group and sum the products. This value is designated as $\Sigma(n_i - 1)s_i^2$. For the example, this is

$$19(13.484) + 19(12.147) + 19(19.882) + 19(21.945)$$
$$+ 19(21.776) + 19(26.892) = 2206.394$$

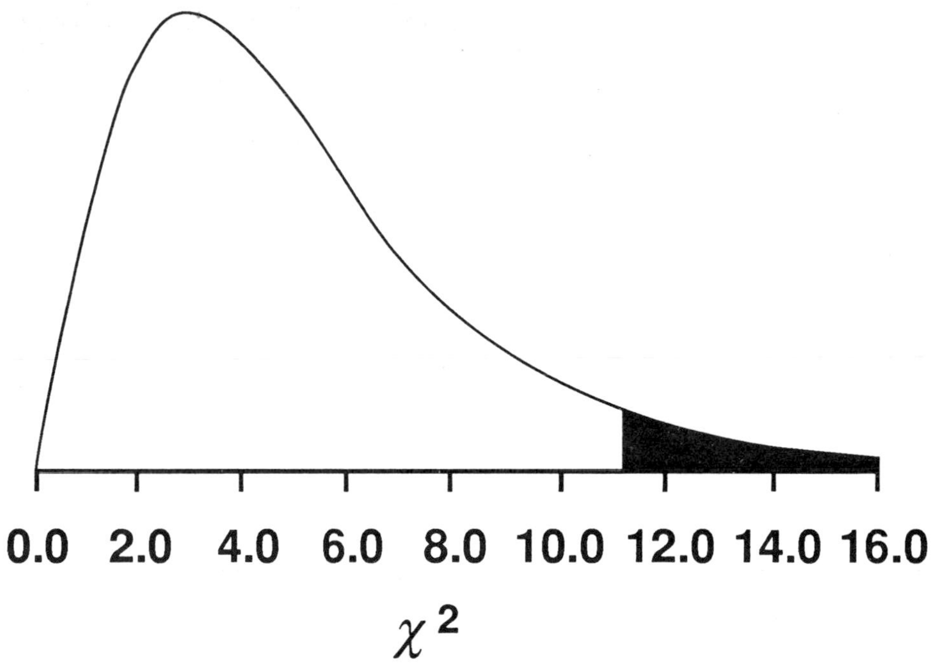

Figure 7.4
A chi-square distribution.

4. Determine the weighted average variance, s_w^2, by

$$s_w^2 = \frac{\Sigma(n_i - 1)s_i^2 \text{(from step 3)}}{\Sigma(n_i - 1) \text{ (from step 2)}}$$

For the example, this value is

$$\frac{2206.394}{114} = 19.354$$

5. Take the natural logarithm of s_w^2. This is designated as $ln\ s_w^2$. For the example, this is

$$ln(19.354) = 2.963$$

6. For each group multiply the degrees of freedom by the natural logarithm of the variance for that group (example 7.8). This value is designated as $\Sigma(n_i - 1)ln\ s_i^2$. For the example, this is

$$19(2.602) + 19(2.497) + 19(2.990) + 19(3.089)$$
$$+ 19(3.080) + 19(3.292) = 333.45$$

Substituting these values in equation 7.16 gives

$$\chi^2 = (114 \times 2.963) - 333.45 = 4.332$$

We now consult table A.3, "Critical Values of the Chi-Square Distribution," for alpha = 0.05 and groups minus 1 degrees of freedom ($6 - 1 = 5$). The critical value is 14.07. Since this value is much larger than our calculated value, we are unable to reject H_0 and conclude that the variances are not unequal.

C A U T I O N

There are a number of important assumptions of ANOVA, one of which is that the within-groups (error) variances of the various groups are all the same. ANOVA is said to be robust to the assumption of normality, meaning that some departure from this assumption is not too serious, particularly when large samples are involved.

When the variable is not even approximately normally distributed and/or when the error variances of the group are unequal, a transformation might correct the problem. Transformations are discussed on the following pages.

When either of these assumptions are not satisfied by the data or when measurement is on an ordinal scale, one should consider one of the nonparametric ANOVAs discussed later in this chapter. In no case should a parametric ANOVA be used with ordinal or nominal data! As mentioned earlier, the error introduced by using a discrete variable is not large provided that the number of values the variable can assume is fairly large.

TRANSFORMATIONS IN ANOVA

There are situations in which the data collected in an experiment do not meet the assumptions of a parametric ANOVA, even though measurement is on an interval or ratio scale and the variable in question is continuous. Two common problems are that the error variances are not equal or that the variable is not approximately normally distributed. Sometimes it is possible to correct one or both of these situations by a **transformation,** which simply involves performing the same mathematical operation on each observation in a set of data. In the following sections, some common transformations and their uses are discussed. For convenience, original observations are designated by the usual x, and transformed observations are designated by x'.

The Logarithmic Transformation

The logarithmic transformation is often useful in ANOVA and in linear regression (see chapter 8) where the error variances are not equal (remember, this is an important assumption in ANOVA, and as we shall see in the next chapter, in linear regression as well). The log transformation is conducted by taking the logarithm of each observation, or

$$x' = \log(x) \tag{7.17}$$

Natural logarithms or base 10 logarithms are commonly used. When there are zeros in the data, one may be added to each observation before taking the log, or

$$x' = \log(x + 1) \tag{7.18}$$

since $\log(0)$ is undefined.

The Square Root Transformation

When data are in the form of frequency counts, a square root transformation often helps improve normality of distribution and/or equality of variances among groups. This transformation involves taking the square root of each observation, or

$$x' = \sqrt{x} \tag{7.19}$$

The Arcsine Transformation

Percentages and proportions tend to be not quite normally distributed, although the underlying variable with which they deal might be, since proportions range from 0 to 1 and percentages range from 0 to 100. Thus, the "tails" of such a distribution tend to be compressed. This situation is noticeable when many of the observations fall below 30% (0.3) or above 70% (0.7). This problem can often be rectified by an arcsine (sine^{-1}) transformation, which, for proportions, is

$$x' = \text{arcsine } \sqrt{x} \tag{7.20}$$

or for percentages is

$$x' = \text{arcsine } \sqrt{\frac{x}{100}} \tag{7.21}$$

Other Transformations

The log transformation, the square root transformation, and the arcsine transformation are perhaps the most commonly used transformations, but they by no means exhaust the list of possibilities.

NONPARAMETRIC ALTERNATIVES TO ANOVA

When data are measured on an ordinal scale, or when data are measured on an interval or ratio scale but the assumptions for parametric ANOVA are not otherwise met, one may use a nonparametric test to compare 3 or more groups. These tests are often called nonparametric ANOVA tests, but since we do not measure variance in nonparametric tests, the name is a bit misleading. In effect, these tests tell us if it is reasonable to assume that 3 or more samples could have been drawn from identical populations.

The Kruskal-Wallis One-way ANOVA

The Kruskal-Wallis one-way ANOVA is the nonparametric counterpart of the completely randomized design. It is used to test the null hypothesis that 3 or more independent samples were drawn from identical populations.

EXAMPLE 7.9   The Kruskal-Wallis One-way ANOVA

The time (in seconds) that males of a certain species of grasshopper remained mounted on females during mating was determined. Ten males each were randomly assigned to 1 of 4 treatments (conditions). The data are as follows.

Treatment A	Treatment B	Treatment C	Treatment D
9	30	3,900	5
3	30	10,800	9
10	480	28,900	20
200	900	3,600	180
1	2	200	15
2	1	120	20
21	5,400	500	2
720	1,500	600	17
1,500	480	1,980	30
60	3	160	8

Modified data from R. Bland

The means and medians for the 4 treatments (conditions) are

	Treatment A	Treatment B	Treatment C	Treatment D
$\bar{x}$	252.6	882.6	5076.0	30.6
m	15.5	255	1290	16

■

Although the experiment is properly designed for a completely randomized ANOVA, and the data are measured on a ratio scale, there are a couple of assumptions of the parametric test that these data do not satisfy. First, the variable does not seem to be even approximately normally distributed, as indicated by the large differences in the means and the medians of each group. As you will recall from chapter 5, the mean and median in a normal distribution are the same, and in samples drawn from such populations one would expect that these 2 values would be at least close to each other. Secondly, the within-groups variances are not equal. Accordingly, we will use the Kruskal-Wallis one-way ANOVA.

Assumptions of the Test

1. The sampled populations have the same but unspecified distribution with the possible exception that one or more of the sampled populations tends to have larger values than one or more of the others.

2. The samples represent random samples from their respective populations.

3. Measurement is on at least an ordinal scale.

4. The samples are from *independent* populations.

To conduct the test, all of the observations in all of the groups are ranked with respect to each other, with the lowest value in any of the samples receiving the rank of one. Tied values receive the average rank that they would have if they were not tied, as in previous examples. The ranked data and the sum of ranks for each group for the example are as follows.

Group A	Group B	Group C	Group D
10.5	19	37	8
6.5	19	39	10.5
12	27.5	40	15.5
25.5	32	36	24
1.5	4	25.5	13
4	1.5	22	15.5
17	38	29	4
31	33.5	30	14
33.5	27.5	35	19
21	6.5	23	9
ΣR 162.5	208.5	316.5	132.5

The test statistic used in the Kruskal-Wallis test is designated as H, which, when the null hypothesis that all of the samples were drawn from identical populations is true, has a chi-square distribution. H is computed by

$$H = \frac{12}{n_t(n_t + 1)}\left(\Sigma\frac{(\Sigma R_i)^2}{n_i}\right) - 3(n_t + 1) \qquad (7.22)$$

where n_i = number of observations in a group, ΣR_i = the sum of ranks in a group, and n_t = the sum of the observations in all of the groups.
For the example

$$H = \frac{12}{40(40 + 1)}\left(\frac{(162.5)^2}{10} + \frac{(208.5)^2}{10}\right.$$
$$\left. + \frac{(316.5)^2}{10} + \frac{(132.5)^2}{10}\right) - 3(40 + 1)$$

$$H = [0.0073 \times (2640.625 + 4347.225 + 10017.225$$
$$+ 1755.625)] - 123 = 13.953$$

H has a chi-square distribution with (groups $-$ 1) df. Consulting table A.3, we find that our calculated value of H is greater than the critical value of chi-square with 2 df at the 0.05 level. We may reject H_0 and conclude that the 3 samples could not have been drawn from identical populations.

The Friedman Two-way ANOVA

The Friedman two-way ANOVA tests whether 3 or more *related* samples could have been drawn from identical populations. Thus, the Friedman two-way ANOVA is equivalent to the randomized complete blocks design.

To conduct the test, the data are arranged in a two-way table of k columns, representing the treatments, and n rows, representing the blocks.

EXAMPLE 7.10   The Friedman Two-Way ANOVA

Do neonatal garter snakes exhibit a decremental response (habituation) to a repeated overhead stimulus? Six snakes were chosen at random and were placed in the experimental chamber and allowed to acclimate for approximately 30 minutes. An overhead rapidly moving object was then presented at 10-second intervals, and the reaction of the snake was noted. Reactions were scored from 3 (a rapid retreat from the stimulus), through 0, which indicated no response.   ∎

These are ordinal data. Since each animal was tested repeatedly, the observations are related and not independent. The data of the experiment are shown in table 7.13.

Table 7.13   Data for Example 7.10

Snake Number (Block)	Interval (Treatment) 1	2	3	4	5	6	7	8
1	3	3	2	2	0	1	0	0
2	3	2	0	2	0	1	0	0
3	2	0	0	0	3	0	0	0
4	2	2	0	0	0	0	0	0
5	3	0	2	0	2	0	0	0
6	2	2	0	1	1	1	1	0

Data from R. Hampton and J. Gillingham

To conduct the test, the observations in each row are ranked with respect to each other (but not with respect to other rows). In other words, each row is ranked independently of the others. Table 7.14 shows the ranked data from table 7.13 with the sums of the columns, which we will use to compute the test statistic.

Table 7.14   Ranked Data for Example 7.10 (from Table 7.13)

Snake Number	Interval 1	2	3	4	5	6	7	8
1	7.5	7.5	5.5	5.5	2	4	2	2
2	8	6.5	2.5	6.5	2.5	5	2.5	2.5
3	7	3.5	3.5	3.5	8	3.5	3.5	3.5
4	7.5	7.5	3.5	3.5	3.5	3.5	3.5	3.5
5	8	3	6.5	3	6.5	3	3	3
6	7.5	7.5	1.5	4.5	4.5	4.5	4.5	1.5
ΣR	45.5	35.5	23	26.5	27	23.5	19	16

The logic of this test is that if there were no difference among the treatments (columns), the sums of the ranks of the columns would be approximately equal. This is because any rank would be as likely to occur in any column as in any other. The test statistic is designated as χ^2_r (chi-square-sub-r) and is given by

$$\chi^2_r = \frac{12}{nk(k+1)}\left[\Sigma(\Sigma R_i)^2\right] - 3n(k+1) \qquad (7.23)$$

where

$$n = \text{number of rows (replicates)}$$
$$k = \text{number of groups (treatments)}$$
$$\Sigma R_i = \text{the sum of ranks of a column}$$

For the example

$$\chi^2_r = \frac{12}{6 \times 8 \times 9} (2070.25 + 1260.25 + 529 + 702.25 + 729$$
$$+ 552.25 + 361 + 256) - (3 \times 6 \times 9) = 18.88$$

When n and k are not too small, χ^2_r has a chi-square distribution. We may therefore consult table A.3 to determine if the differences among the 8 treatments are significant. The degrees of freedom in the Friedman test are $k - 1$, which, for the example, is $8 - 1 = 7$. The critical value of chi-square at alpha $= 0.05$ with 7 degrees of freedom is 14.07. Since our calculated value of χ^2_r is greater than this, we may reject the null hypothesis that there is no significant difference between the treatments. Since, in this case, "treatments" are the successive presentations of the test stimulus at 10-second intervals, we conclude that neonatal garter snakes exhibit a decremental response (habituate) to the stimulus.

COMPUTER SUPPLEMENT

Figure 7.5 shows the MINITAB-generated ANOVA table for example 7.2, the means and their confidence intervals, and a graphic representation of the means and their confidence intervals.

The MINITAB-generated ANOVA table for example 7.5, showing the brooding time of male convict cichlids, is shown in figure 7.6. Note that the command for the randomized complete blocks design is different than the completely randomized design of example 7.2.

Finally, the MINITAB-generated ANOVA table for example 7.7, a factorial design, is given in figure 7.7. Again, note that the command for this design is distinct from that of the other designs.

```
:MTB > aovoneway c1-c6
:
:ANALYSIS OF VARIANCE
:SOURCE       DF           SS        MS         F        p
:FACTOR        5       1585.5     317.1     16.38    0.000
:ERROR       114       2206.4      19.4
:TOTAL       119       3791.9
:                                    INDIVIDUAL 95 PCT CI'S FOR MEAN
:                                    BASED ON POOLED STDEV
:  LEVEL       N         MEAN     STDEV    -+---------+---------+---------+-----
:lakea        20       33.700     3.672     (----*-----)
:lakeb        20       33.400     3.485    (----*-----)
:lakec        20       34.250     4.459     (-----*----)
:streama      20       42.050     4.685                            (----*-----)
:streamb      20       40.250     4.667                        (-----*-----)
:streamc      20       40.550     5.186                        (-----*----)
:                                          -+---------+---------+---------+-----
:POOLED STDEV =        4.399              31.5      35.0      38.5      42.0
:MTB >
```

Figure 7.5
MINITAB printout for example 7.2.

```
:Analysis of Variance for time
:
:Source      DF           SS         MS        F       P
:day          4       513502     128375    24.23   0.000
:male         7       215601      30800     5.81   0.000
:Error       28       148334       5298
:Total       39       877437
:
:
:      MEANS
:
: day    N         time
:  1     8        40.29
:  2     8        65.16
:  3     8       194.26
:  4     8       292.56
:  5     8       316.46
:
:MTB >
```

Figure 7.6
MINITAB printout for example 7.5.

```
MTB > anova c3=c1 c2 c1*c2;
SUBC> means c1 c2 c1*c2.

Factor       Type Levels Values
sex          fixed    2     1       2
location     fixed    3     1       2       3

Analysis of Variance for length

Source          DF         SS         MS        F       P
sex              1      511.58     511.58    26.41   0.000
location         2      335.94     167.97     8.67   0.001
sex*location     2      350.84     175.42     9.06   0.000
Error           54     1046.03      19.37
Total           59     2244.39

      MEANS

sex     N      length
 1     30      56.477
 2     30      50.637

location    N      length
   1       20      50.830
   2       20      56.600
   3       20      53.240

sex location    N      length
 1      1       10      56.120
 1      2       10      56.200
 1      3       10      57.110
 2      1       10      45.540
 2      2       10      57.000
 2      3       10      49.370
```

Figure 7.7
MINITAB printout for example 7.7.

between-groups
 variance (treatment
 variance)
completely random
 design ANOVA with
 fixed effects
 (model I)
error variance (within-
 groups variance)
experimental data

factorial design
interaction
multiple comparisons
observational data
random-effects (model
 II) ANOVA
randomized complete
 blocks design
transformation

For the following problems, assume that the variable is approximately normally distributed unless instructed otherwise. For each problem identify the ANOVA design involved, state the null hypothesis or hypotheses, and construct an ANOVA table. Conduct a multiple-comparisons test if appropriate to the specific problem. State a biological conclusion based on your statistical analysis. Where appropriate, construct a graphic interpretation. (Exercises preceded by an asterisk are suitable for a computer solution.)

Exercises 7.1 through 7.10 are the completely randomized design. Assume normality of distribution and equality of variances.

7.1   Fifteen tobacco plants of the same age and genetic strain were randomly assigned to 3 groups of 5 plants each. One group was untreated, one was infected with tobacco mosaic virus (TMV), and one was infected with tobacco ringspot virus (TRSV). After one week the activity of *o*-diphenol oxidase was determined in each plant. Does infection by either virus affect the activity of this enzyme?

Enzyme Activity (μl O_2/mg protein/min)		
Control	TMV-Infected	TRSV-Infected
1.47	2.44	2.87
1.62	2.31	3.05
1.06	1.98	2.36
0.89	2.76	3.21
1.67	2.39	3.00

7.2   Eighteen freshwater clams were randomly assigned to 3 groups of 6 each. One group was placed in the pond water from which the clams were collected, one group was placed in deionized water, and one group was placed in a solution of 0.5 mM sodium sulfate. At the end of a specified time period, blood potassium levels were determined. Do the treatments affect blood potassium levels?

	$\mu M\ K^+$	
Pond Water	Deionized Water	Sodium Sulfate
.518	.318	.393
.523	.342	.415
.495	.301	.351
.502	.390	.390
.525	.327	.385
.490	.320	.397

Data from J. Schiede

7.3 Cellulase activity in 4 genetic variants of a fungus species was measured in 5 randomly selected cultures of each variant. Is there a difference in activity of this enzyme in the 4 variants?

	Enzyme Activity (units/mg protein) in		
Variant A	Variant B	Variant C	Variant D
10	20	15	5
12	21	18	3
9	19	13	6
11	23	14	6
10	18	12	4

7.4 Forty adult mice of a highly inbred laboratory strain were randomly assigned to 5 groups of 8 each in a controlled environment in which the lights were on from 7 A.M. until 7 P.M. and off from 7 P.M. until 7 A.M. After several weeks plasma sodium concentration was determined for one group at each of the times indicated in the data table. Does time of day influence plasma sodium concentration?

	Plasma Na$^+$ (meq/liter)			
	Light		Dark	
7 AM	1 PM	7 PM	1 AM	7 AM
148	138	140	137	143
152	130	138	135	152
150	132	129	148	149
149	129	140	140	150
160	140	142	137	161
155	139	139	141	155
162	130	132	145	149
149	142	141	136	162

Data from J. Schiede

7.5 Fifteen juniper pythons of similar size and age were randomly assigned to 3 groups. One group was treated with drug A, one group with drug B, and the third group was not treated. Their systolic blood pressure was measured 24 hours after administration of the treatments. Does either drug affect blood pressure? Does one have more or less of an effect than the other?

Drug A	Drug B	Untreated
118	105	130
120	110	135
125	98	132
119	106	128
121	105	130

7.6 Thirty pea seeds were randomly assigned to 3 groups of 10 each. One group was germinated in the presence of chemical A, a second group was germinated in the presence of chemical B, and the third group served as a control. After 5 days the length (in millimeters) of the primary root was measured. We wish to know if either or both of these chemicals affects root growth, and if so, if one is more effective than the other.

Chemical A	Chemical B	Control
115	120	82
103	125	97
98	122	105
121	100	90
130	90	102
107	128	98
106	121	105
120	115	89
100	130	100
125	120	90

7.7 Random samples of a certain species of zooplankton were collected from 5 randomly selected lakes and their selenium content was determined. We wish to know if there is a difference among lakes with respect to selenium content in this species (i.e., is there a significant "lake effect"?).

Lake A	Lake B	Lake C	Lake D	Lake E
23	34	15	18	25
30	42	18	15	20
28	39	12	9	22
32	40	10	12	18
35	38	8	10	30
27	41	16	17	22
30	40	20	10	20
32	39	19	12	19

7.8 Twenty-seven chickens were randomly assigned to 3 groups of 9 each. One group was fed chicken feed containing 1 ppb of a pesticide, a second group feed containing 100 ppb of the pesticide, and the third group feed containing none of the pesticide (control). Unfortunately, one of the animals in the 1 ppb group escaped and has not been seen since. After 6 weeks with these diets, SRBC antibody titers of the animals were determined. Is there an effect of the pesticide at either concentration?

1 ppb	100 ppb	Control
5	9	7
8	10	11
5	11	12
12	9	9
11	13	8
6	10	11
7	11	8
5	10	9
6		10

7.9   An experiment similar to the one described in exercise 7.8 was conducted. In this case 4 randomly selected groups of 9 chickens each were given feed containing 1 of 3 randomly selected insecticides, and their *Brucella abortus* antibody titers were measured. We wish to know if exposure to insecticides affects the immune response to *B. abortus* (a bacterial pathogen of chickens) in chickens.

Insecticide A	Insecticide B	Insecticide C	Control
15	11	9	10
12	9	11	8
18	8	8	9
12	8	11	10
17	10	9	11
11	8	8	9
12	9	10	9
13	10	9	11
15	8	9	8

7.10   Fifteen turkey hens were randomly assigned to 3 groups of 5. One group was given diet A, the second group diet B, and the third group diet C. We wish to know if there is a difference in the weight of eggs produced by the birds on these diets, and if so, which diet results in the largest eggs. The data are the mean weights of 10 eggs from each bird.

Diet A	Diet B	Diet C
124	98	116
118	100	97
120	95	100
127	102	89
115	105	98

Exercises 7.11 through 7.20 are the randomized complete blocks design. Assume normality of distribution, equality of variances, and absence of interaction.

7.11   Three mice from each of 6 litters were randomly assigned to 3 treatment groups. One group was exposed to 100 ppb methyl mercury, one group was exposed to 100 ppb mercuric chloride, and the third group served as a control. The time (in minutes) that each mouse spent on an exercise wheel in one day was measured several days after exposure. Does exposure to mercury cause the animals to be more or less active, and if so, is there an effect of the chemical form of the mercury?

Litter Number	Methyl Mercury	Mercuric Chloride	Control
1	60	90	50
2	100	120	80
3	40	45	35
4	120	110	100
5	80	105	60
6	130	155	105

7.12   An investigator wished to test the effect of 3 diets on the parastalic blood pressure of mangrove toads. Because these animals are rare, only a few may be collected in any one location. Three toads were collected from each of 5 locations and one toad from each location was randomly assigned to one of the 3 diets. Is there a difference in blood pressure that is related to the 3 diets?

Location	Diet A	Diet B	Diet C
1	65	75	80
2	60	69	79
3	55	50	70
4	53	54	80
5	64	69	85

7.13   Photosynthesis in 5 tobacco plants was measured before, one day after, and one week after exposure at a temperature of 100°F for 2 hours. We wish to know if exposure to this temperature affects the rate of photosynthesis, and if so, if the rate of photosynthesis returns to its pretreatment level within one week.

Plant Number	Photosynthesis (μM $CO_2/min/g$)		
	Before Treatment	One Day After Treatment	One Week After Treatment
1	127	107	130
2	130	111	127
3	240	222	250
4	116	98	120
5	215	201	200

7.14   Males of the Northern water snake apparently court females at the expense of time spent foraging. Thus, the energetic "cost" of courtship, if any, might be measured as weight loss in males through the short mating season. Five marked male Northern water snakes were captured, weighed, and released at the beginning, near the middle, and at the end of the mating season. Using the data given in the following table, determine if there was a significant weight loss in males during this period. (Experiment suggested by H. Carbone.)

	Weight (in grams) at		
Snake Number	Beginning	Middle	End
1	397	362	325
2	410	385	350
3	362	325	300
4	291	270	253
5	325	289	280

7.15 Testosterone levels in 6 captive male bush hogs was measured at 4 times during the year. The mating season for this species occurs in the fall. Do the data below support the hypothesis that testosterone levels in this species are higher during the mating season?

	Plasma Testosterone Level			
Male Number	Winter	Spring	Summer	Fall
1	20	30	25	220
2	30	20	70	210
3	40	90	50	230
4	35	40	40	190
5	60	60	105	100
6	55	40	72	210

7.16 Three hens from each of 3 varieties were randomly assigned to 3 diets. We wish to determine if there is a difference in egg weight produced by the 3 diets, and if so, which diet produces the largest eggs. The data are the mean weights of 10 eggs from each bird.

	Mean Egg Weight With		
Variety	Diet A	Diet B	Diet C
1	112	87	100
2	100	82	98
3	90	75	86

7.17 A parcel of land was divided into 6 equally sized plots (blocks), and each block was divided into 3 equally sized subplots. Three treatments (no added nitrogen, 10 lbs nitrogen/hectare, and 100 lbs nitrogen/hectare) were randomly assigned to the subplots within each plot. Does added nitrogen increase the growth of a certain crop? Data are pounds of yield per subplot.

	Crop Yield With		
Block	No added N	10 lbs/hectare	100 lbs/hectare
1	105	156	187
2	98	145	167
3	125	170	201
4	100	150	180
5	130	185	210
6	80	135	162

7.18   The concentration of unicellular algae (measured as chlorophyll concentration per liter) at 3 different depths in 4 lakes was measured. We wish to know if there is a difference in algae concentration that is related to depth. Lakes are treated as blocks to take into account differences among lakes.

Lake	Surface	1 m	3 m
1	425	130	56
2	500	215	115
3	100	30	10
4	325	100	28

7.19   A plant ecologist wished to determine if an exotic weed might be becoming more numerous in a particular area. She randomly selected 5 one-meter-square quadrates in the area of interest and counted the number of individual plants of the weed in each quadrate over a period of 5 years. Is there a significant increase in this species over this time period?

Quadrate Number	Year				
	1	2	3	4	5
1	2	5	8	10	20
2	5	9	17	30	40
3	15	30	31	60	72
4	0	2	9	15	24
5	9	11	23	17	45

7.20   Six rug rats were given a small amount of caffeine. Their pulse rate was measured before, immediately after, and one hour after administration of the caffeine. Does caffeine affect pulse rate in this species?

Rat Number	Pulse Rate		
	Before	Immediately After	One Hour After
1	105	115	108
2	98	110	100
3	110	125	115
4	100	112	105
5	114	130	120
6	90	100	95

Exercises 7.21 through 7.26 are the factorial design. Assume normality of distribution and equality of variances.

7.21 The effect of infection by tobacco mosaic virus (TMV) and tobacco ringspot virus (TRSV) on *o*-diphenol oxidase activity in 3 genetic strains of tobacco was measured. The results are given in the following data table.

	Treatment		
	Noninfected	TMV-infected	TRSV-infected
Strain A	102	237	117
	115	219	95
	98	201	128
Strain B	97	193	105
	85	175	60
	63	160	91
Strain C	127	230	135
	150	249	145
	168	250	170

Answer the following questions and support your answers with the appropriate ANOVA.

7.21a Does virus infection affect this enzyme?

7.21b Is there a difference in the activity of this enzyme among strains?

7.21c Do different strains respond differently to virus infection (i.e., is there a significant interaction between the 2 main effects?)?

7.21d Show the results graphically.

7.22 The possible influence of crowding and sex on plasma corticosterone in a highly inbred strain of rug rats was investigated using a factorial design. Sex (males, nongravid females, and gravid females) and crowding (low, moderate, and high) were used as the main treatment effects. The results were as follows.

	Crowding		
Sex	Low	Moderate	High
Males	5	115	253
	8	122	249
	13	119	260
	9	130	257
	15	114	280
	11	129	263
Nongravid Females	12	112	219
	19	115	222
	15	121	218
	20	117	220
	11	118	223
	18	120	225
Gravid Females	37	157	289
	42	160	273
	50	173	280
	35	182	291
	40	168	205
	36	170	296

Write a paragraph or two discussing the results given above from a biological perspective, and support your conclusions with the proper statistical analysis. Include a graphic representation of the effects of these 2 factors and any possible interaction between them.

7.23 Forty-five large female guppies were randomly assigned to 9 groups, each of which received different amounts of food and were kept at different temperatures in a two-way factorial design. The number of offspring that each produced in a single brood are given in the following table. We wish to know if there is an effect of temperature, an effect of food intake, and an interaction of these 2 factors on the number of offspring per brood produced by these animals.

Temperature	Number of Daily Feedings		
	1	2	3
70°F	18	25	28
	20	30	36
	15	19	29
	27	30	30
	30	25	37
75°F	20	28	33
	28	29	39
	30	32	42
	17	38	47
	29	29	38
80°F	35	35	51
	30	39	42
	32	30	48
	28	40	39
	35	38	55

7.24 The possible effects of sex and age on systolic blood pressure in hamsters was investigated, with the following results. Determine if there is an effect of sex, an effect of age, and an interaction of these 2 factors.

Age	Sex	
	Male	Female
Adolescent	108	110
	110	105
	90	100
	80	90
	100	102
Mature	120	110
	125	105
	130	115
	120	100
	130	120
Old	145	130
	150	125
	130	135
	155	130
	140	120

*7.25 Using the data from table B.3 (see appendix B), determine if there is an effect of smoking, an effect of sex, and an interaction between these 2 on pulse rate in humans.

*7.26 Using the data from table B.3, determine if reaction time is different between males and females, athletes and nonathletes; also determine if there is an interaction between sex and participation in a varsity sport.

7.27 Using the data from exercise 7.1, determine if the error variances may be considered to be equal.

7.28 Using the data from exercise 7.2, determine if the error variances may be considered to be equal.

7.29 Using the data from exercise 7.3, determine if the error variances may be considered to be equal.

7.30 Using the data from exercise 7.4, determine if the error variances may be considered to be equal.

7.31 Using the data from exercise 7.5, determine if the error variances may be considered to be equal.

7.32 Using the data from exercise 7.6, determine if the error variances may be considered to be equal.

7.33 Using the data from exercise 7.36, determine if the error groups variances may be considered to be equal.

7.34 Using the data from exercise 7.37, determine if the error groups variances may be considered to be equal.

Exercises 7.35 through 7.40 are appropriate for the Kruskal-Wallis one-way ANOVA.

7.35 Fifteen inbred laboratory rats were randomly assigned to 3 groups of 5 each. Each rat was inoculated with *Staphylococcus mucans,* a bacterium involved in the process of tooth decay. One group (control) was given no additional treatment. A second group was given drug A, and a third group was given drug B. At the end of 6 weeks, the extent of tooth decay in the rats was evaluated as percent of tooth decay. This is a fairly subjective measurement based on the combined evaluation of 3 observers and should probably be regarded as an ordinal measurement. We wish to know if there is a difference among the 3 groups.

	Percent of Decay in	
Control	Drug A	Drug B
87	63	45
76	70	60
65	87	43
81	92	56
75	70	60

Conduct the appropriate test and state a conclusion.

7.36 Thirty chickens of a highly inbred strain were randomly assigned to 3 groups of 10. One group was injected with 100 μg norepinephrin per kilogram of body weight, a second group was injected with 100 μg epinephrin per kilogram of body weight, and a third group served as the control. SRBC plaque forming cells per 10^6 spleen cells were measured after a specified time interval. The variances among the 3 groups are not equal, and the variable may or may not be normally distributed. Is there a difference among the 3 groups?

Norepinephrin	Epinephrin	Control
15	70	535
155	45	370
110	95	420
90	95	315
35	70	485
100	315	230
30	140	370
40	260	320
75	230	335
105	400	475

7.37 Testosterone levels in mature roosters of 3 strains of chickens were measured, and the following results were obtained. It appears that the variances within the groups are unequal, and we do not know if the variable is normally distributed. Is there a difference among strains?

Strain A	Strain B	Strain C
439	102	107
568	115	99
134	98	102
897	126	105
229	115	89
329	120	110

7.38 The aggressiveness of 15 randomly selected female gully cats was measured under 3 different conditions. Aggressiveness was measured on a rather subjective scale of 0 to 100 and should be regarded as an ordinal measurement. We wish to know if there is a difference in aggressiveness among the 3 conditions. The results were as follows.

Condition A	Condition B	Condition C
5	20	60
10	15	50
20	20	70
8	25	25
11	27	90

7.39 Three groups of eggs of a tropical frog were exposed to either water containing no benzene (control group), water containing 50 ppm benzene, and water saturated with benzene. After hatching, the brain size of the froglets was measured. We wish to determine if exposure to benzene affects brain size. We do not know if this variable is approximately normally distributed, nor is it possible to determine its distribution with a sample as small as this. The results were as follows.

Control	50 ppm	Saturated
81	88	111
72	89	109
68	92	133
87	107	
	101	
	91	

Data from J. Martin

7.40 Twenty-four rug rats were randomly assigned to 4 groups of 6 each. The groups were subjected to different levels of stress (high, moderate, low, and none) induced by playing rap music for them. After one week, blood lymphocytes (cells $\times 10^6$/ml) were measured. We do not know if this variable is normally distributed in this species.

High	Moderate	Low	None
2.9	3.7	5.2	6.8
1.8	4.6	6.2	7.9
2.1	4.2	5.7	7.1
1.5	2.8	4.6	6.5
0.9	3.2	5.1	6.3
2.8	4.5	4.9	7.6

Exercises 7.41 through 7.46 are appropriate for the Friedman two-way ANOVA.

7.41 Six male mosquito fish were selected at random from a large population. Each was placed individually in an aquarium with a female, and the number of copulatory attempts made during 5 successive three-minute intervals was recorded. The results were as follows.

Male Number	Interval Number				
	1	2	3	4	5
1	20	10	7	5	2
2	18	7	5	5	3
3	25	13	9	4	1
4	10	5	3	2	1
5	12	15	8	3	0
6	17	4	5	2	1

We wish to know if males exhibit a diminishing response (habituate) to individual females.

7.42 Six damsel fly naiads were placed individually into 6 containers, which contained 10 each of 4 different prey species. After a short time, the number of each prey species eaten was recorded. Is there a preference for any of the prey items? (Experiment suggested by J. Havel.)

Naiad Number	Prey A	Prey B	Prey C	Prey D
1	8	3	1	2
2	9	5	4	1
3	7	1	0	0
4	10	7	8	1
5	8	9	1	2
6	9	2	1	3

7.43   Three randomly selected mice from each of 6 litters were randomly assigned to 3 treatment groups. One group received injections of 100 ug/kg of epinephrin, the second group received injections of 100 ug/kg of norepinephrin, and the third group served as a control. SRBC antibody titers were measured one week after treatment. The variable does not appear to be normally distributed, nor are the error variances equal.

Litter Number	Epinephrin	Norepinephrin	Control
1	125	180	350
2	225	112	400
3	180	290	375
4	300	225	495
5	115	325	427
6	98	115	510

7.44   Using the data from exercise 7.16, suppose we doubt that the variable is approximately normally distributed. Conduct the appropriate test, and state a conclusion.

7.45   Conduct an appropriate nonparametric test using the data from exercise 7.15, and state a conclusion.

7.46   Conduct an appropriate nonparametric test using the data from exercise 7.17, and state a conclusion.

Correlation and Regression

Often in biological research we are interested in exploring the possible relationships between 2 or more variables. Some examples of such relationships are the relationship between age and blood pressure, the size of females of certain species and the number of offspring they produce, the relationship between the dosage level of some drug and a particular physiological response, and so on. In all of these cases, 2 variables are measured for each individual in our sample, and we seek to detect a relationship between these 2 variables.

In this chapter we will consider statistical techniques designed to detect such relationships between 2 variables measured on at least an ordinal scale. In the following chapter, we will consider how to deal with associations between variables measured on a nominal scale. The techniques we will consider here are correlation and simple linear regression. Which of these techniques is used for any particular problem depends on the nature of the data collected and on the nature of the questions being asked about the data.

Correlation is used to determine (1) if an association between 2 variables exists, and (2) how strong such an association is. By association, we mean that as one variable changes, the other changes in some consistent way. Note that in the case of correlation, there is no assumption about a "cause-and-effect" association between the 2 variables, although such a relationship might exist. For example, we might wish to know if the size of a female iguana is associated with the number of eggs she produces (see example 8.1). Size and number of eggs are both approximately normally distributed variables, and they may or may not be related in some way. The number of eggs a female produces is not the "cause" of her size, and conversely, her size is not necessarily a "cause" of the number of eggs she produces (although size might be an important contributing factor in determining the number of eggs). Both variables may, in fact, be under the control of a third variable, such as age or nutrition. If well-fed females tend to be large because of the amount of food they obtain, and if they also produce more eggs because of the amount of food they obtain, then size and number of eggs produced by a female are related, but both variables are under the control of a third variable: nutrition, in this case.

Regression analysis, on the other hand, traditionally assumes a cause-and-effect relationship between the 2 variables, such that at least a substantial proportion of the variation in one of the variables, called the **dependent variable,** can be explained by or attributed to the other variable, called the **independent variable.**

For example, we might wish to investigate a possible relationship between caffeine consumption and pulse rate. We can assume that, if such a relationship exists, it is the amount of caffeine consumed (the independent variable) that causes a change in pulse rate (the dependent variable), and not the other way around.

Another important distinction between correlation and regression is that in the most common type of regression analysis, the independent variable is usually not a normally distributed random variable; rather, it is under the control of the investigator. In this respect regression as it is usually done is a fixed-effects (model I) design similar to a fixed-effects ANOVA. In effect this means that the experimenter chooses what levels of caffeine to administer to the test subjects in our example. A random-effects design, analogous to a random-effects ANOVA (see chapter 7), may be used with regression analysis. However, this is quite uncommon, and we will not consider the details of this procedure.

Regression analysis may be extended to include more than one independent variable acting on a dependent variable, a technique known as multiple linear regression. However, our treatment here will be limited to simple linear regression, in which only one independent and one dependent variable is considered.

Judging from the biological research literature, there seems to be a good deal of confusion about when one should use correlation and when one should use regression analysis. Some statisticians make a fairly rigid and clear-cut distinction between these 2 techniques, particularly with regard to the types of data to which they may be applied, while other statisticians, and apparently many biologists, seem to take a much more relaxed attitude about the whole affair and use the 2 approaches almost interchangeably. Examples 8.1, 8.2, and 8.3 will help to clarify the distinction between correlation and regression.

EXAMPLE 8.1   A Correlation Problem

Data from a random sample of 11 gravid female iguanas including their postpartum weight and the number of eggs each produced, were collected. The results are given in table 8.1, and the scattergram for these data is shown in figure 8.1. ◾

We will arbitrarily designate weight as the x variable and the number of eggs as the y variable. In a correlation analysis, which, as we shall later see, is the proper treatment for a problem of this sort, it makes no difference which variable is plotted on which axis, as long as we are consistent from one observation to the next.

Table 8.1   Postpartum Weight of Female Iguanas and Number of Eggs Produced

Specimen Number	Mass (in Kilograms)	Number of Eggs
1	0.90	33
2	1.55	50
3	1.30	46
4	1.00	33
5	1.55	53
6	1.80	57
7	1.50	44
8	1.05	31
9	1.70	60
10	1.20	40
11	1.45	50

Data from T. Miller

A cursory examination of the data in table 8.1 and figure 8.1 might lead us to suspect that larger females produce more eggs (i.e., that there is a relationship, or correlation, between a female's size and the number of eggs she produces in a single brood).

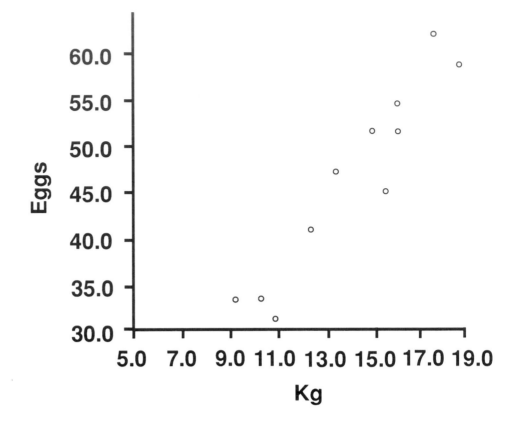

Figure 8.1
Postpartum weight of female
iguanas vs. **number of eggs**
produced (data from example
8.1).

EXAMPLE 8.2 A Regression Problem

A snake physiologist wished to investigate the effect of temperature on the heart rate of juniper pythons. She selected 9 specimens of approximately the same age, size, and sex and placed each animal at a preselected temperature between 2° and 18°C. After the snakes had equilibrated to their ambient temperatures, she measured their heart rates. The results are given in table 8.2. ∎

Note that in this experiment the temperatures were selected, or under the control of the investigator. In this case temperature is not a random variable in the population.

Table 8.2 The Relationship between Temperature
and Heart Rate in Juniper Pythons

Snake Number	Temperature (°C)	Heart Rate (BPM)
1	2	5
2	4	11
3	6	11
4	8	14
5	10	22
6	12	23
7	14	32
8	16	29
9	18	32

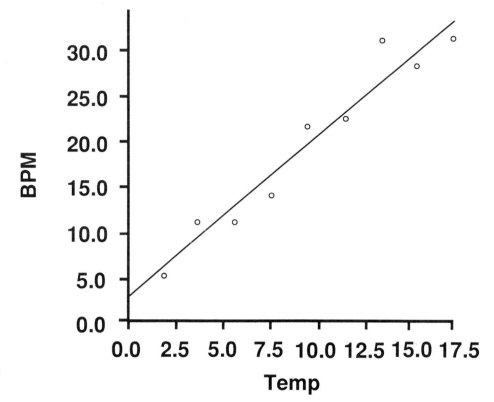

Figure 8.2
Heartbeat rate of juniper
pythons as a function of
temperature (data from example
8.2).

The scattergram for these data is shown in figure 8.2. Note that temperature is plotted on the *x*-axis, and heart rate is plotted on the *y*-axis, and not vice versa. Furthermore, we have drawn a line through the points and could, if we choose, write an equation that describes this line. Using this equation we could even predict the heart rate of juniper pythons at various temperatures.

EXAMPLE 8.3   Another Regression Problem

Suppose in the experiment described in example 8.1 that the investigator had selected a sample of female iguanas based on their weight and determined the number of eggs that they produced. In this case the individuals included in the sample were not chosen at random but rather on the basis of the variable assumed to be the independent variable (i.e., the independent variable is under the control of the investigator in this case).   ∎

Provided that we are willing to assume that the number of eggs that a female produces is at least partially "caused" or influenced by her weight, and if the intent is to write an equation that will allow a prediction of the number of eggs a female might produce based on her weight, we would treat this situation as a regression problem. To some extent the procedure used depends on the question being asked, and it always depends on the design of the experiment. In example 8.1, which is an example of a situation applicable to the correlation model, female iguanas were sampled at random. In example 8.3 they were selected on the basis of their size, and therefore, size is not a random variable.

The first example is a proper problem for correlation analysis, while the second and third examples are proper problems for regression analysis. While the 2 examples appear to be very much alike and to ask the same basic question (i.e., is there a relationship between the 2 variables?), there are many important differences between these 2 situations. In the first example, gravid female iguanas were selected at random from a population. The 2 variables measured (postpartum weight and number of eggs produced) are assumed to be normally distributed variables in the population, and neither was controlled by the investigator. With data like these, we do correlation analysis, and we should resist the temptation to conduct the more sophisticated regression analysis!

In the second and third examples, the investigator selected the values of the independent variable (always designated as the *x* variable) to be used in the experiment, and therefore, in neither case is the independent variable treated as a random variable in the population. In both cases the dependent variable (designated as the *y* variable) is assumed to be at least partially under the control of the independent variable. In situations like these, regression analysis is the proper treatment of the data.

CORRELATION

In correlation analysis, we ask 2 questions: (1) Are 2 variables related in some consistent and linear way?, and (2) What is the strength of the relationship? The strength of such relationships refers to how closely the points in a scattergram of the data cluster about an imaginary line drawn through them. (Note that we do not actually draw this line, and it would be improper to do so in a correlation analysis.)

The Pearson Correlation Coefficient

The measure of the strength of the relationship between 2 variables in a correlation is the **correlation coefficient.** When our data are measured on an interval or ratio scale, when both variables are approximately normally distributed, and when certain other assumptions, discussed below, are met, we may use the Pearson correlation coefficient (sometimes called the product moment correlation coefficient). This parameter of the population is designated by the Greek symbol rho (ρ). Usually, the true value of this parameter is unknown to us, and we must estimate its value from a random sample of the population. The sample correlation coefficient, which is used to estimate the parametric correlation coefficient, is designated as *r*. The value of ρ (or *r*) ranges from $+1$, indicating a perfect positive correlation; through 0, indicating no relationship between the 2 variables; to -1, indicating a perfect negative correlation between the 2 variables. The sample correlation coefficient, *r,* is not a measure of significance of the relationship. It is, once again, a measure of the strength of the relationship. A low value for *r* indicates a weak relationship, which may nevertheless be "real," or significant.

The null hypothesis in a correlation analysis is that the parametric correlation coefficient, ρ, is zero, or

$$H_0: \rho = 0$$

When we are able to reject H_0, we conclude that ρ is not equal to zero and that therefore a correlation or association between the two variables exists.

Assumptions of the Test

1. The sample is a random sample from the population of interest.
2. Both variables are approximately normally distributed.
3. Measurement of both variables is on an interval or ratio scale.
4. The relationship between the 2 variables, if it exists, is linear.

When assumption 2 is not met, transformation (see chapter 7) of one or both variables may make them approximately normally distributed. However, great care must be taken here, since a transformation may cause the relationship to be nonlinear, and thus, assumption 4 would be violated. When assumptions 2 and/or 3 and/or 4 are not met, one of the nonparametric correlation tests discussed later in this chapter should be used. When assumption 4 is not met, transformation of one or both variables (see chapter 7) might make the relationship linear. Again though, caution should be exercised here, since transformation to make the relationship linear may result in a nonnormal distribution. When assumption 1 is not met, a new sample must be collected.

We will use example 8.1 (see p. 153), concerning the relationship between the postpartum weight of female iguanas and the number of eggs they produce in a single brood, to illustrate the calculations involved in correlation analysis. These data are reproduced in table 8.3 with some preliminary calculations and are shown graphically in figure 8.1.

Table 8.3   Postpartum Weight of Female Iguanas and Number of Eggs Produced

Specimen Number	Mass (in Kilograms)	Number of Eggs
1	0.90	33
2	1.55	50
3	1.30	46
4	1.00	33
5	1.55	53
6	1.80	57
7	1.50	44
8	1.05	31
9	1.70	60
10	1.20	40
11	1.45	50

$$\Sigma x = 15 \qquad \Sigma y = 497$$
$$\Sigma x^2 = 21.33 \qquad \Sigma y^2 = 23{,}449$$
$$(\Sigma x)^2 = 225 \qquad (\Sigma y)^2 = 247{,}009$$
$$\Sigma xy = 705.8$$
$$\Sigma x \Sigma y = 7{,}455$$

In this example, the data are measured on a ratio scale, and both variables may be assumed to be approximately normally distributed. Accordingly, we may compute the Pearson correlation coefficient. The computational techniques in computing the sample correlation coefficient (r), from which we estimate the parametric correlation coefficient (ρ), are mostly familiar to you by now from ANOVA. The sample correlation coefficient is given by

$$r = \frac{\Sigma xy - \dfrac{\Sigma x \Sigma y}{n}}{\sqrt{\left(\Sigma x^2 - \dfrac{(\Sigma x)^2}{n}\right)\left(\Sigma y^2 - \dfrac{(\Sigma y)^2}{n}\right)}} \qquad (8.1)$$

The value Σxy is the only calculation that we have not encountered before. It is obtained by multiplying each x value by its corresponding y value and summing the products. The numerator in equation 8.1 is called the covariance, and it measures how x and y vary together. You will recognize the denominator as the square root of the product of the sums of squares of the x and y variables. Substituting the values from the example in equation 8.1 gives

$$r = \frac{705.8 - \left[\dfrac{(15)(497)}{11}\right]}{\sqrt{\left(21.33 - \dfrac{(15)^2}{11}\right)\left(23{,}449 - \dfrac{(497)^2}{11}\right)}} = 0.952$$

Testing the Significance of r

The correlation coefficient is a measure of the strength of the relationship between 2 variables; it is not a test of the significance of the relationship, although many people seem to treat it this way. A value of r near one, as we obtained in the previous example, indicates a strong relationship, while a low value of r indicates a weak relationship. Neither of these is necessarily more "significant," in a statistical sense, than the other. Although a relationship may be weak, as indicated by a low value of r, it may nevertheless be quite significant.

Recall that the null hypothesis in a correlation analysis is that p, the population correlation coefficient, is zero. The sample correlation coefficient, r, is an estimate of this population correlation coefficient. When the null hypothesis is that the population correlation is zero (the usual case), r has a t distribution with $n - 2$ degrees of freedom. We calculate t by

$$t = r \sqrt{\frac{n - 2}{1 - r^2}} \qquad (8.2)$$

For the example,

$$t = 0.952 \sqrt{\frac{9}{1 - 0.906}} = 9.315$$

The critical value of t for alpha $= 0.05$ and 9 df is 2.262 for a two-tailed probability. We may therefore reject the null hypothesis and conclude that the 2 variables are correlated.

An alternative way of determining if r is significant is to consult table A.8, "Critical Values of the Pearson Correlation Coefficient (r)." This table gives the minimum values of r that permit one to reject the null hypothesis. If the calculated value of r is equal to or greater than the tabular value for the specified degrees of freedom $(n - 2)$, the null hypothesis is rejected.

Nonparametric Correlation Analysis (Spearman's r)

When data are measured on an ordinal scale, or when other assumptions of the parametric correlation test just discussed are not met, one may use one of several nonparametric correlation tests. The most commonly used of these is the Spearman rank correlation test. The assumptions of this test are that observations are a random sample from the population and that measurement of both variables is at least ordinal.

EXAMPLE 8.4   A Nonparametric Correlation

The mass (in grams)·of 13 adult male tuatara and the size of their territories (in square meters) was measured. Are territory size and the size of the male holding the territory related (i.e., do larger males hold larger territories?)? ■

Mass of these animals is probably approximately normally distributed, but it seems doubtful that the area of their territories is, and even if it were, territory size is rather difficult to measure accurately. For these reasons a nonparametric correlation test seems to be in order. The results were as follows (we arbitrarily designate mass as the x variable and territory size as the y variable).

Table 8.4   Mass and Territory Size of Adult Male Tuataras

Observation Number	Mass (x)	Rx	Territory Size (y)	Ry	d	d²
1	510	6	6.9	6	0	0
2	773	9	20.6	11	−2	4
3	840	13	17.2	9	4	16
4	505	5	6.7	5	0	0
5	765	8	20.0	12	−4	16
6	780	10	24.1	13	−3	9
7	235	1	1.5	1	0	0
8	790	11	13.8	8	3	9
9	440	3	1.7	2	1	1
10	435	2	2.1	3	−1	1
11	815	12	20.2	10	2	4
12	460	4	3.0	4	0	0
13	697	7	10.3	7	0	0

$$\Sigma d^2 = 60$$

Data from J. Gillingham

The steps involved in calculating the Spearman correlation coefficient, r_s, follow. We will use the tuatara data (table 8.4) as an example.

1. Rank the observations in the x variable from smallest to largest. These are designated as Rx in the table.
2. Rank the observations in the y variable from smallest to largest. These are designated as Ry in the table. (Note: The x and y variables are ranked separately.)

3. Subtract each Ry from its corresponding Rx (designated as d in the table), and square each difference (designated as d^2).
4. Sum the values of d^2, which is designated as Σd^2. For the example, this value is 60.
5. Calculate r_s using equation 8.3.

$$r_s = 1 - \left(\frac{6\Sigma d^2}{n(n^2 - 1)}\right) \tag{8.3}$$

where n is the number of observations.
For the example,

$$r_s = 1 - \left(\frac{6 \times 60}{13(169 - 1)}\right) = 0.835$$

Testing the Significance of r_s

The null hypothesis in the Spearman correlation test is essentially the same as it is for the Pearson (parametric) test, which is that there is no relationship between the 2 variables. We may test the significance of r_s by using equation 8.2 in the same manner that the significance of the Pearson correlation coefficient was tested. For the example,

$$t = 0.835 \sqrt{\frac{13 - 2}{1 - (0.835)^2}} = 4.89$$

If our computed value of t is equal to or greater than the critical value of t for the desired level of alpha at $n - 2$ degrees of freedom (see table A.2), we may reject H$_0$.

The null hypothesis may also be tested by consulting table A.9. This table gives minimum values of r_s, which are significant at various degrees of freedom. When the calculated value of r_s is equal to or greater than the table value, the null hypothesis is rejected.

SIMPLE LINEAR REGRESSION

Regression is similar to correlation analysis in some respects, except that in regression analysis we usually assume that there is a cause-and-effect relationship between the 2 variables under study and that the independent variable is under the control of the investigator (i.e., that a fixed-effects experimental design is used). In effect, we hypothesize that there is a functional relationship that permits us to predict a value of the dependent variable, y, corresponding to a given value of the independent variable, x. Mathematically, such a relationship is expressed as

$$y = f(x)$$

In simple linear regression, this relationship takes the form

$$\mu_y = \alpha + \beta x$$

where μ_y is the population mean value of y at any value of x, α is the population intercept and β is the population slope.

Regression analysis has several uses, which include but are not limited to the following.

1. Regression is used to approximate an equation that describes the linear relationship between the 2 variables in question. This is called

the **regression equation** or the regression function. Since the parameters α and β are usually unknown to us, we estimate these values from a sample.

2. From this equation we are able to construct a line through the points of a scattergram, which is called the **regression (least squares) line.**

3. The regression equation may be used to predict values of the dependent variable (y) at various values of the independent variable (x).

4. Regression may be used to estimate the extent to which the dependent variable is under the control of the independent variable.

Regression analysis is based on several assumptions. Unless these assumptions are met, one should either use correlation analysis, if the assumptions of those tests are met, or redesign the experiment.

Assumptions of the Test

1. The independent variable is fixed. This means, in effect, that values of the independent variable are chosen by the investigator and do not represent a random variable in the population. There is no variance associated with the independent variable!

2. For any value of the independent variable (x), there exists a normally distributed population of values of the dependent variable, y. The population mean of these values of y, μ_y is

$$\mu_y = \alpha + \beta x$$

where α is the population intercept and β is the population slope of the regression equation.

3. It follows from assumption 2 that for any value of x, any particular value of y is

$$y_i = \alpha + \beta x + e$$

In this case, e, called a **residual,** is the amount by which any observed value of y differs from the mean value of y. These residuals (sometimes called error terms) have a standard normal distribution.

4. The variances of the y variable for all values of x are equal.

5. Observations are independent. This means that each individual in the sample is measured only once!

Some of these assumptions are rather obscure, but their meanings should become clear as we proceed. When assumption 1 is not met, regression is not the proper treatment for the data, but correlation might be.

Consider the imaginary experiment to determine the relationship, if any, between temperature and heart rate in juniper pythons (example 8.2). The investigator selected a series of temperatures (assumption 1) and designated this as the independent variable. She then placed a different animal at each of the preselected temperatures and measured its heart rate (the dependent variable). The data obtained in the experiment are shown in table 8.5.

Table 8.5 The Effect of Temperature on the Heart Rate of Juniper Pythons

Temperature (°C) (x)	Heart Rate (y)
2	5
4	11
6	11
8	14
10	22
12	23
14	32
16	29
18	32
$\Sigma x = 90$	$\Sigma y = 179$
$\overline{x} = 10$	$\overline{y} = 19.88$

Note that the investigator measured only one individual at each temperature (this is all that is necessary) and that at each temperature a different individual was used (assumption 5). Had she measured the heart rate of one individual at different temperatures, the observations would not have been independent. The data in table 8.5 are plotted as a scattergram in figure 8.2. Note that, although not all of the points seem to fall on a straight line, there seems to be a definite linear relationship between the 2 variables (assumption 2, in part). What can regression tell us about this relationship?

Estimating the Regression Function and the Regression Line

One of the things we are interested in doing with regression analysis is to estimate the parametric regression function (regression equation), $\mu_y = \alpha + \beta x,$ where α is the intercept and β is the slope of the equation. We estimate these values using a sample. The estimated intercept is designated as a and the estimated slope, usually called the **regression coefficient,** is designated as b. The line described by this equation is the line that best "fits" the regression function, and it is called the estimated regression line. Since the line and the equation are one and the same (the equation defines the line), we will be considering them together in the following few sections. There is one point through which the regression line always passes, and that is the point defined by $\overline{x}, \overline{y}$. In figure 8.3 a horizontal line has been placed through this point. A vertical line has been constructed from each value of y to this horizontal line. Each of these vertical lines represents the amount by which the observed value of y deviates from the mean value of y, or

$$y - \overline{y}$$

The sum of these $y - \overline{y}$ values is approximately 0 (see table 8.6). However, if we square each of these $y - \overline{y}$ and then sum them, or

$$\Sigma(y - \overline{y})^2$$

we would have a sum of squares for y. Note that this value is large (see table 8.6).

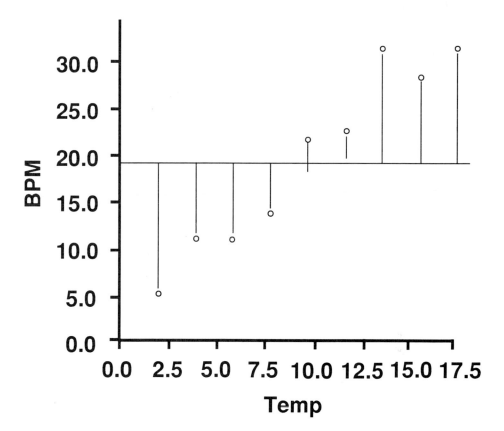

Figure 8.3
Graphic representation of the
variation in dependent variable
when independent variable is
not considered.

Table 8.6 Data from Table 8.5

x	y	$y - \bar{y}$	$(y - \bar{y})^2$	$\hat{y}$	$e\ (y - \hat{y})$
2	5	−14.89	221.71	5.69	−0.69
4	11	− 8.89	79.03	9.24	1.76
6	11	− 8.89	79.03	12.79	−1.79
8	14	− 5.89	34.69	16.33	−2.34
10	22	2.11	4.45	19.89	2.11
12	23	3.11	9.67	23.44	−0.44
14	32	12.11	146.65	26.99	5.01
16	29	9.11	82.99	30.54	−1.54
18	32	12.11	146.65	34.09	−2.09
	Σ	− 0.01	804.87	$\Sigma(y - \hat{y})^2 =$	48.74

Before terminal confusion sets in, we will review what we have just done here. In effect, we have calculated a sum of squares for y without taking x (temperature) into account. In other words, we can see that there is a great deal of variance in heart rate among our 9 subjects when we do not consider their temperature.

Suppose now that we could rotate the line in figure 8.3, using $\bar{x}, \bar{y}$ as a pivot, until it is in a position such that the deviations of the y values from this line were minimized, or more specifically, in a position such that the sum of

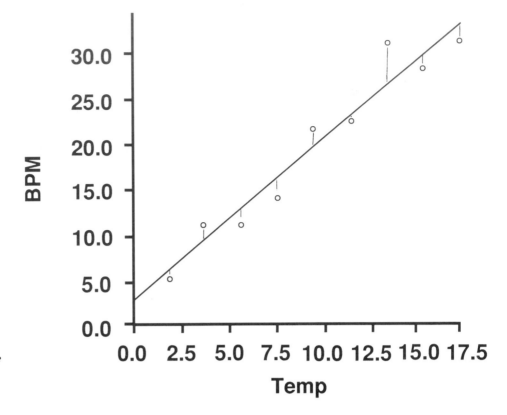

Figure 8.4
Graphic representation of the variation in dependent variable when independent variable is considered.

the squares of the deviations of the y values from the line were minimized (see figure 8.4). Such a line would best "fit" our data. You will note that the observed values of y do not all fall on this line (sometimes none of them do). This is the regression line. We will see later how it is calculated. That value of y that would fall exactly on this line, as described by the regression equation, is referred to as $\hat{y}$ ("y hat"). As before, we have constructed vertical lines from each value of y to this new line, and these vertical lines have the value

$$y - \hat{y}$$

These values, given in table 8.6, represent the amount by which each observed value of y deviates from the regression line. For the moment do not be concerned with how we defined the regression line or how the values of $\hat{y}$ were calculated. We will return to this later. Squaring the values of $y - \hat{y}$ in table 8.6 and then summing them gives us another sum of squares for y. This sum of squares represents the variance in y when temperature (x) is taken into account. Note that it is much smaller than the variance in y when x was not considered. In statistical jargon, we have decreased the uncertainty of y by considering x. What does this mean exactly?

If we were given information regarding the heartbeat rate of these 9 juniper pythons in our example but had no knowledge of their temperatures, and if from these data we were asked to predict something about the heartbeat rate of juniper pythons, we could only conclude that the mean heartbeat is around 19.89 BPM with a great deal of variation from animal to animal (estimated from $(y - \bar{y})^2$, which is large). On the other hand, given a knowledge of x (temperature), we could make a much more accurate prediction of the heartbeat rate of juniper pythons.

Refer once again to table 8.6 and figure 8.4. Note that the values y do not coincide with the values of $\hat{y}$. The amount by which y and $\hat{y}$ differ (given in the column designated e in table 8.7) is called a residual and is denoted by the symbol e. One of the assumptions of regression is that the residuals are normally distributed with a mean of zero (assumption 3, in part).

Calculating the Estimated Regression Equation

The estimated slope of the regression equation is given by

$$b = \frac{\Sigma xy - \dfrac{\Sigma x \Sigma y}{n}}{\Sigma x^2 - \dfrac{(\Sigma x)^2}{n}} \tag{8.4}$$

The estimated intercept is given by

$$a = \bar{y} - b\bar{x} \tag{8.5}$$

For the juniper python example (table 8.5),

$$b = \frac{2216 - \dfrac{16110}{9}}{1140 - \dfrac{8100}{9}} = 1.775$$

and

$$a = 19.89 - (1.775 \times 10) = 2.14$$

The estimated regression function is therefore

$$\hat{y} = 2.14 + 1.775x$$

The regression line is defined by the values of $\hat{y}$ corresponding to values of x. The regression line may be constructed graphically by plotting the values of $\hat{y}$ versus the corresponding values of x. We have now obtained estimates of the slope of the regression equation (b), the y-intercept (a), and the regression line. We now need to attach some statistical significance to these estimates.

Table 8.7   The Effect of Temperature on the Heart Rate of Juniper Pythons

Temperature (°C) (x)	Heart Rate (y)	$\hat{y}$	e (Residual)
2	5	5.69	−0.69
4	11	9.24	1.76
6	11	12.79	−1.79
8	14	16.33	−2.34
10	22	19.89	2.11
12	23	23.44	−0.44
14	32	26.99	5.01
16	29	30.54	−1.54
18	32	34.09	−2.09
$\Sigma x = 90$	$\Sigma y = 179$	$\Sigma(y - \bar{y})^2 = 804.89$	
$\bar{x} = 10$	$\bar{y} = 19.89$	$\Sigma(y - \hat{y})^2 = 48.74$	
$\Sigma x^2 = 1140$	$\Sigma y^2 = 4365$		
$(\Sigma x)^2 = 8100$	$(\Sigma y)^2 = 32041$		
$\Sigma x\bar{y} = 2216$	$\Sigma x \Sigma y = 16110$		

Testing the Significance of the Regression Equation

Recall that the sample slope, b, is an estimate of the parametric slope, β. Even if $\beta = 0$, which would indicate no dependence of y on x, we might expect b to occasionally have a nonzero value by chance alone. We therefore test the null hypothesis $H_0: \beta = 0$. We will use an ANOVA technique for this test. To conduct the ANOVA, we need 3 sums of squares and their associated degrees of freedom: the total sum of squares with $n - 1$ degrees of freedom, the regression sum of squares with one degree of freedom, and the error sum of squares with $n - 2$ degrees of freedom. Table 8.7 gives the values needed to calculate these sums of squares.

The total sum of squares, $\Sigma(y - \bar{y})^2$, is given by

$$SS_t = \Sigma y^2 - \frac{(\Sigma y)^2}{n} \tag{8.6}$$

This is sum of squares for y when x is not considered.
For the example,

$$SS_t = 4365 - \frac{32041}{9} = 805$$

The regression sum of squares is given by

$$SS_r = b\left(\Sigma xy - \frac{\Sigma x \Sigma y}{n}\right) \tag{8.7}$$

This is the sum of squares for y when x is considered.
For the example,

$$SS_r = 1.775\left(2216 - \frac{16110}{8}\right) = 756.15$$

The error sum of squares is given by

$$SS_e = SS_t - SS_r \tag{8.8}$$

This is the sum of squares of the residuals, and it represents the variance in y that is still present when x is considered. In other words, it is the error sum of squares.
For the example,

$$SS_e = 805 - 756.15 = 48.85$$

The ANOVA table is constructed as before (see table 8.8).

Table 8.8 ANOVA Table for the Data in Table 8.7

Source	SS	df	MS	F
Regression	756.15	1	756.15	108.33
Error	48.85	7	6.98	
Total	805.00	8		

The critical value of F for 1 and 7 df at $\alpha = 0.05$ is 5.59. Thus, we reject $H_0: \beta = 0$ and conclude that the value of y is dependent on the value of x (i.e., that the regression slope is not zero).

The Confidence Interval for β

Recall that b is an estimate of β, the regression coefficient. As usual, we cannot say that $\beta = b$, but we can compute a 95% confidence interval for β. The standard error for b, s_b, is given by

$$s_b = \sqrt{\frac{MS_e}{\Sigma x^2 - \frac{(\Sigma x)^2}{n}}} \tag{8.9}$$

where MS_e is the mean square for error (from the ANOVA table). The confidence interval for β is then

$$\beta = b \pm s_b\,(t_{0.05,\,n-2}) \tag{8.10}$$

where t is the two-tailed probability of t at alpha $= 0.05$ with $n - 2$ degrees of freedom.

For the example,

$$s_b = \sqrt{\frac{6.98}{1140 - \frac{8100}{9}}} = 0.1705$$

then

$$\beta = 1.775 \pm 0.1705 \times 2.365$$

gives the upper and lower confidence limits for b, which are

$$2.178 > \beta > 1.371$$

The Coefficient of Determination (r^2)

We know that the variance in y is greatly reduced by a knowledge of x, but there is usually still some variance remaining in y when x has been considered (the error variance). If the value of y were completely dependent on x, there would be no error variance, which is to say that all of our observations would fall on the regression line. We may properly ask, "What proportion of the variance in y is explained by its dependence on x?" To determine this, we compute the **coefficient of determination, r^2**. This value is computed by

$$r^2 = \frac{SS_r}{SS_t} \tag{8.11}$$

For the example,

$$r^2 = \frac{756.15}{805} = 0.939$$

Thus, we may conclude that 0.939 or 93.9% of the variance in y is dependent on x, which is to say that when we know the value of x, we reduce the uncertainty about y by 93.9%. Note that there is a residual or "unexplained" variance of $100 - 93.9 = 6.1\%$ of the variance in y that is still not explained. This is the variance among individuals that is not related to x. We will return to this unexplained variance later.

The coefficient of determination may also be computed for a correlation analysis, in which case it is the square of the correlation coefficient, r. However, in correlation treatments, r^2 should not be considered as a measure of the variation in y that is explained or dependent upon x, but rather as the variation in y that is *associated* with the variance of x, and vice versa.

Predicting y from x

One important use of regression is to enable us to predict a value of y for a given value of x. This must be done with some restraint, however. In the juniper python example, we measured heart rate (y) for temperatures (x) between 2°C and 18°C. Predictions about heart rate well beyond these measured values (called extrapolation) may or may not be meaningful. For example, we would predict a very high heart rate at 100°C by using the regression function, but biologically we would probably predict a heart rate of zero! In a similar manner we would probably predict a negative heart rate at temperatures much below zero, which is clearly silly!

Even when predictions about y are kept within reasonable limits of x, it is important to remember that y is usually not an exact function of x, since y is a normally distributed random variable. Thus, when we predict a value of y from x, what we are in fact doing is estimating the population mean value of y for any particular value of x. This estimated value is designated as $\hat{y}$. As usual, we should affix confidence limits to this estimate.

To continue with the juniper python example, we wish to know the mean heart rate of all juniper pythons at 15°C. First, we calculate the value of $\hat{y}$ at $x = 15$ degrees from the regression equation, which is

$$\hat{y} = 2.14 + (1.775 \times 15) = 28.77$$

We now compute the standard error of y, which is given by

$$s_{\hat{y}} = \sqrt{\mathrm{MS}_e \left[\frac{1}{n} + \frac{(x - \overline{x})^2}{\Sigma x^2 - \frac{(\Sigma x)^2}{n}} \right]} \tag{8.12}$$

where x is that value of x for which we wish to have a confidence interval for y, and $\overline{x}$ is the mean value of x. For the example,

$$s_{\hat{y}} = \sqrt{6.98 \left[\frac{1}{9} + \frac{(15 - 10)^2}{240} \right]} = 1.228$$

The 95% confidence interval for the predicted mean value of y at 15°C is

$$\mu_{\hat{y}} = \hat{y} \pm s_{\hat{y}} \, t_{(0.05, \, n - 2)}$$

where t is the tabular value of t at alpha 0.05 and $n - 2$ degrees of freedom. For the example,

$$\mu_y = 28.77 \pm (1.228 \times 2.365) = 28.77 \pm 2.904$$

or

$$31.67 > \mu_y > 25.87$$

We conclude that there is a probability of 0.95 that these limits include the population value μ_y at 15°C. A graphic representation of the confidence in-

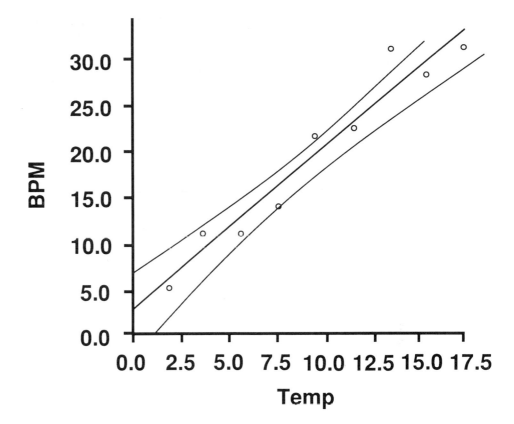

Figure 8.5
The 95% confidence interval
(prediction interval) for
example 8.2.

terval (or prediction interval) of μ_y at various values of x is shown in figure 8.5. The lines above and below the regression line show the 95% prediction interval for μ_y at any value of x within our measured limits of x. Note that the prediction interval becomes wider at lower and higher values of x.

Dealing with Several Values of y for Each Value of x

Frequently, data that are to be analyzed by regression are conducted as we have outlined previously. Note that in our example, there is only one value of y for each value of x, which is to say that only one snake was measured at each temperature. For various reasons, it is sometimes desirable or necessary to measure the value of the dependent variable, y, for several individuals at each value of the independent variable, x. For example, an investigator might wish to test only a few values of x. Using only one measurement of y at each x would result in a sample size that might be too small to reveal a significant association (i.e., a sample size that would result in a high probability of a type II error).

EXAMPLE 8.5 More Than One Value of y for Each Value of x

For purposes of illustration, we will redesign the juniper python experiment somewhat, this time using only 3 temperatures but measuring the heart rate of several snakes at each temperature. The results of the experiment are given in table 8.9. ■

*Table 8.9   The Effect of Temperature
on the Heart Rate of Juniper Pythons
(Several Values of y for Each x)*

Temperature	Heart Rate
4	9
4	8
4	11
4	8
10	20
10	21
10	19
10	20
10	19
10	20
16	30
16	28
16	31
16	29
16	30

With the data arrayed in this way, we may proceed exactly as before when there was only one value of y for each value of x. Note carefully, however, that the sum of x is not $4 + 10 + 16$; rather it is $(4 \times 4) + (6 \times 10) + (5 \times 16)$. In other words, we do not have 3 values of x—we have 15, some of which are the same! The scattergram for these data, showing the regression line and the 95% prediction interval, is given in figure 8.6.

C A U T I O N

In the example we have just examined, 15 snakes were used. It is sometimes tempting to measure the same individual repeatedly at each value of x, which, in our example, would be only 3 snakes. This is a serious violation of independence (see chapter 1). Had we done the experiment in this way, we could use the mean value of y at each x as a datum (which is sometimes a useful thing to do), but our sample size would be 3, not 15.

Transformations in Regression

When the relationship between the variables in a regression analysis does not seem to be linear (assumption 2), it is sometimes possible to make the relationship linear by transforming one or both of the variables (see chapter 7).

COMPUTER SUPPLEMENT

Simple linear regression using most current statistical packages is relatively straightforward. The MINITAB printout for example 8.2 (the effect of temperature on the heart rate of juniper pythons) is shown in figure 8.7. Note that all of the values we calculated for the examples are included in the printout. In addition, several statistical packages, including MINITAB, enable one to test various assumptions of linear regression.

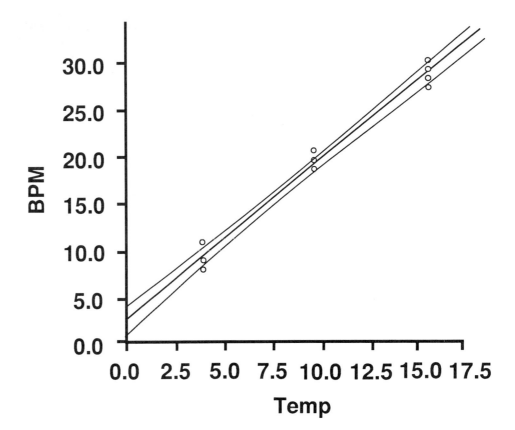

Figure 8.6
The 95% confidence interval
(prediction interval) for
example 8.5.

```
MTB > brief 3
MTB > regress 'hbr' 1 'temp'

The regression equation is
hbr = 2.14 + 1.77 temp

Predictor       Coef      Stdev     t-ratio        p
Constant        2.139     1.917       1.12      0.301
temp            1.7750    0.1703     10.42      0.000

s = 2.639       R-sq = 93.9%      R-sq(adj) = 93.1%

Analysis of Variance

SOURCE        DF          SS          MS         F        p
Regression     1       756.15      756.15    108.60    0.000
Error          7        48.74        6.96
Total          8       804.89

Obs.    temp       hbr       Fit  Stdev.Fit  Residual   St.Resid
  1      2.0     5.000     5.689     1.622     -0.689     -0.33
  2      4.0    11.000     9.239     1.348      1.761      0.78
  3      6.0    11.000    12.789     1.113     -1.789     -0.75
  4      8.0    14.000    16.339     0.943     -2.339     -0.95
  5     10.0    22.000    19.889     0.880      2.111      0.85
  6     12.0    23.000    23.439     0.943     -0.439     -0.18
  7     14.0    32.000    26.989     1.113      5.011      2.09R
  8     16.0    29.000    30.539     1.348     -1.539     -0.68
  9     18.0    32.000    34.089     1.622     -2.089     -1.00

R denotes an obs. with a large st. resid.
```

Figure 8.7
MINITAB printout for example 8.2.

KEY TERMS

coefficient of
   determination
correlation coefficient
dependent variable
independent variable

regression coefficient
regression equation
regression (least
   squares) line
residual

EXERCISES

For exercises 8.1 through 8.14, compute the sample correlation coefficient, test the null hypothesis $\rho = 0$, and draw the scattergram of the data. Assume a bivariate normal distribution. (Exercises preceded by an asterisk are suitable for a computer solution.)

8.1 A random sample of twenty-eight sexually mature female garter snakes was collected. Among other things, the snout-vent length (in centimeters) and the weight (in grams) of each snake was measured. Is there an association between length and weight?

Snake Number	Length	Weight
1	44.5	96
2	49.0	68
3	41.0	72
4	30.0	17
5	48.0	94
6	43.0	52
7	41.0	74
8	53.0	92
9	52.0	92
10	50.0	64
11	49.5	80
12	49.0	86
13	48.5	52
14	44.0	71
15	50.5	87
16	48.5	85
17	50.5	69
18	68.5	214
19	52.0	152
20	42.0	83
21	42.0	90
22	46.0	59
23	52.0	92
24	70.5	170
25	58.5	120
26	50.5	94
27	40.5	53
28	48.0	51

8.2 A random sample of female mosquito fish was collected. Their total length and the number of embryos that each contained were determined. Is there an association between length and number of embryos?

Length	Number of Embryos	Length	Number of Embryos
30	19	32	35
28	8	33	17
53	59	34	39
39	56	30	25
37	23	34	38
37	27	33	19
37	26	32	17
37	52	30	17
39	59	32	26
36	31	32	16
33	19	29	18
35	50	30	22
38	53	31	21
39	22	36	17
30	9	33	20

8.3   The age, systolic blood pressure, and diastolic blood pressure for a random sample of people were determined. Is there a correlation of age and systolic blood pressure?

Age	Systolic	Diastolic	Age	Systolic	Diastolic
22	114	74	21	112	68
20	118	68	25	111	70
7	94	54	7	90	53
10	94	48	9	92	56
30	118	64	21	120	70
21	140	70	24	120	80
35	118	78	37	138	84
38	120	80	29	123	78
10	100	40	41	132	83
22	125	90	22	110	77
15	108	58	11	102	66
46	130	90	19	108	74
39	130	94	79	140	86
22	104	62	22	132	72
58	134	72	24	138	82
46	122	86	37	122	78
37	142	82	26	132	64
40	122	62	40	125	63
37	110	72	9	90	42
27	110	64	20	122	78
21	110	68	21	106	62
22	138	82	51	118	78
20	118	62	20	120	78
19	118	76	36	132	76
53	114	78	18	118	80
43	112	78	21	115	70
33	116	79	22	114	70
36	117	78	13	106	66
21	114	76	25	114	66
41	116	74	21	110	70
38	102	62	7	80	42

8.4 Using the data from exercise 8.3, determine if a relationship between age and diastolic blood pressure exists.

8.5 Using the data from exercise 8.3, determine if a relationship between systolic and diastolic blood pressure exists.

8.6 It is likely that students who do well on an examination in a particular course are likely to score well on a subsequent examination in that same course, and that students who do not do well on the first exam are likely to not do well on the second exam (i.e., exam scores on the 2 exams will be correlated). Below are the scores on 2 examinations for 45 randomly selected students in a general biology course. Is there an association between the scores on the two tests?

Test 1	Test 2	Test 1	Test 2	Test 1	Test 2
63	76	49	71	66	67
51	48	46	69	72	57
46	64	54	62	74	74
74	88	74	88	74	83
83	88	40	64	83	83
80	86	74	83	83	86
49	79	72	60	83	83
89	79	72	62	80	57
77	74	51	52	80	62
86	79	66	74	72	50
46	79	89	88	83	69
60	74	60	79	77	60
66	83	74	64	92	88
66	71	72	74	86	74
54	81	69	76	60	62

8.7 Ten randomly selected soil samples were analyzed for krypton content (μg/kg soil) using an old, expensive, but very reliable and accurate method; and a newer, less expensive and faster method. A strong correlation between the results of the 2 methods would indicate that the new method is also accurate.

Old Method	New Method
25	27
30	28
20	19
35	36
40	38
25	25
33	32
50	52
65	67
60	58

8.8 Total body weight, spleen weight, and bursa weight of 9 newly hatched turkeys were determined. Is there a correlation between total body weight and spleen weight?

Body Weight (in grams)	Spleen Weight (in milligrams)	Bursa Weight (in milligrams)
53.81	18.9	50.8
56.26	20.4	51.4
59.86	15.9	28.4
59.96	19.9	66.6
61.75	17.4	35.5
55.28	24.0	38.8
56.57	21.3	50.3
49.91	16.2	33.2
54.25	19.3	39.3

8.9   Using the data from exercise 8.8, determine if there is a significant correlation between total body weight and bursa weight.

8.10   Using the data from exercise 8.8, determine if there is a significant correlation between spleen weight and bursa weight.

8.11   The weight, length, and width of 44 randomly selected killdeer eggs were determined. Is there a correlation between weight and width?

Weight	Width	Length
13	26.4	36.7
13	26.5	36.5
12	26.4	34.3
13.5	27.1	37.1
15.5	28.3	38.1
15	28	37.2
15	28	38.1
14	27.2	37.5
14	27.7	36.7
15	27.6	38.3
14.5	28	36.5
14.5	27.2	39.5
14.5	26.8	39.1
13	26	39.6
13	26	36.9
12.5	27.3	36.4
12	26.7	36
12.5	27.3	36.5
12.5	26.8	37.1
14.5	27.2	37.6
14.5	27.4	39.5
13.5	27.8	38.1
13.5	27.4	37.4
13.5	26.9	38.5
14	27.4	37.8
15.5	28.7	38
15.5	28.4	39
16	28.4	39
12.5	26.3	37.6

(*Continued on p. 176*)

Weight	Width	Length
13	26.5	37.6
12	25.9	37.1
14	27.1	38.3
15	27	42
14.5	27.3	39.6
14	27	37.8
15	27.2	40.2
12	27.5	35.3
12.5	27.3	34.3
13	26.3	38.1
13	26.4	38.2
13	28.3	39.3
14	29.4	38.7
15	28.4	39.6
14	27.7	39.3

Data from D. Blaszkiewicz

8.12 Using the data from 8.11, determine if there is a correlation between weight and length.

8.13 Using the data from 8.11, determine if there is a correlation between length and width.

*8.14 Using the data in table B.3, determine if there is a correlation between pulse rate and reaction time in humans.

For exercises 8.15 through 8.24, compute the regression equation, test the null hypothesis that $\beta = 0$, compute the 95% confidence interval for the slope, compute the coefficient of determination, compute y and the 95% confidence interval for μ_y for each value of x, and graph your results. Answer any additional questions specific to each exercise.

8.15 Algae cells were incubated in a culture medium containing different concentrations of dilithium chloride. After a period of incubation, the concentration of dilithium ($\mu g/g$) in the algae cells was determined.

Concentration in Medium ($\mu M/l$)	Concentration in Cells ($\mu g/g$)
0	0
1	9
2	21
5	47
10	105
20	213

8.16 The cadmium concentration of grasses at different distances from a major highway at randomly selected locations was measured, with the following results.

Distance (in meters)	Cadmium (µg/kg)
1	105
2	48
3	39
4	28
5	18
10	9

8.17   Nine male road warblers of different ages were selected and their systolic blood pressure was measured. (Nine or 10 years is considered very old among road warblers.) The results were as follows.

Age (in years)	Blood Pressure
1	103
2	115
3	109
4	114
5	120
6	119
7	128
8	132
9	138

8.18   The wattle thickness in chickens given 5 concentrations of PHA was as follows.

Concentration	Wattle Thickness (in millimeters)
0	1.01
1	1.53
2	2.00
3	2.47
4	3.01
5	3.66

8.19   The rate of an enzyme catalyzed reaction (*o*-diphenol oxidase) was measured at different substrate concentrations. Rate is the dependent variable. A reciprocal transformation of both variables is required to make the relationship linear.

Substrate Concentration (mM)	Rate (µl O_2/min)
0.20	105.3
0.30	142.9
0.40	166.7
0.50	181.8
1.00	256.4

8.20 Ten colonies of juvenile hamsters were established with different densities of animals ranging from 1 to 5 animals per square meter. After one week 3 animals were randomly selected from each colony and their serum corticosterone was measured. The relationship does not appear to be linear. You might wish to try one or more transformations (chapter 7) to attempt to rectify the situation.

Density	Serum Corticosterone
1	3.2
1	2.8
1	3.1
2	8.5
2	10.2
2	9.9
3	27.5
3	34.0
3	29.8
4	97.2
4	120.0
4	105.6
5	330.0
5	285.0
5	315.5

8.21 Tomato plants of the same genetic strain and age were subjected to a temperature of 115°F for a period of 3 hours. Such treatment reduces the plants' ability to photosynthesize. One plant from the group was randomly selected each day for 11 consecutive days, and its rate of photosynthesis was determined. We wish to know if the plants recover from this temperature stress, and if so, write an equation to describe the rate of recovery. The results were as follows.

Days Posttreatment	Photosynthetic Rate ($\mu M\ CO_2$/gram/sec)
0	15.0
1	17.5
2	16.5
3	19.0
4	22.0
5	24.0
6	22.5
7	26.5
8	25.0
9	30.0
10	29.0

8.22   Garter snakes were trained to not respond to a threat stimulus (habituated). After a specified period of time, the stimulus was again presented and the number of times the snakes responded was recorded. The ratio of the second presentation responses to the first presentation responses was considered to be a measure of memory. Thus, a ratio of zero would indicate complete memory, and a ratio of one would indicate no memory. We wish to write an equation to describe the rate of memory loss.

Interval between Stimulus Presentations (in minutes)	Ratio
4	.20
4	.25
4	.00
4	.09
4	.11
8	.60
8	.20
8	.20
8	.50
8	.39
12	.50
12	.30
12	.29
12	.54
12	.58
16	1.06
16	.58
16	.50
16	.56
16	.77
20	.95
20	.43
20	.50
20	.25
20	.57
24	.57
24	.90
24	.50
24	.92
24	.89

8.23   A certain species of bacterium was cultured in the presence of various concentrations of methyl mercury. The number of cells (per milliliter) in the various cultures was determined after a period of incubation.

Methyl Mercury (μM)	Cells × 10⁶/ml
0	6.6
0	6.9
0	7.2
1	6.8
1	6.0
1	5.6
2	6.4
2	6.0
2	5.4
4	4.8
4	4.4
4	3.9
6	2.6
6	3.1
6	3.4
8	1.0
8	1.3
8	1.7
10	0.2
10	0.3
10	0.5

8.24 Kingfisher nestlings 5 to 7 days old were incubated at different ambient temperatures, and their body temperatures were measured. At this age the birds are not capable of maintaining a constant body temperature as are older birds. The nestlings were randomly assigned to the various temperatures. The results were as follows.

Ambient Temperature (°C)	Body Temperature (°C)
10	10
10	12
10	11
10	17
10	15
10	13
20	21
20	28
20	27
20	27
20	24
20	25
20	20
30	29
30	31
30	28
30	35
30	36
30	30
40	40
40	39
40	35
40	37
40	37
40	40
40	38

Data from M. Hamas

Frequencies and Nominal Data

In many types of biological research, we are interested in the frequencies with which certain events or objects occur, and often the data we collect are measured on a nominal scale. The tests we have considered up to this point are not really suited to the analysis of frequencies or nominal data. In this chapter we will consider several tests designed to deal with frequency counts and/or nominal data.

THE CHI-SQUARE (χ^2) GOODNESS OF FIT TEST

We are often interested in determining if a frequency distribution of a sample from a population fits or does not fit some expected theoretical distribution, such as a Poisson, binomial, or normal distribution—or for that matter, any sort of distribution we care to specify. Several tests, called **goodness of fit tests,** are designed for this purpose.

The null hypothesis for a goodness of fit test is that an observed frequency distribution is not different from some specified distribution and that any departure of the frequency distribution of the sample from the specified distribution is therefore due to chance alone.

Chances are that you are already acquainted with the chi-square goodness of fit test from genetics. The chi-square goodness of fit test does exactly what its name indicates: it tests how well a set of observed frequencies in 2 or more mutually exclusive categories fit (or do not fit) some specified (expected) distribution. It is a nonparametric test and requires only nominal measurement or other frequency counts.

Assumptions of the Test

1. Measurement is on at least a nominal scale. Categories of the nominal scale or of the groups whose frequencies are represented are mutually exclusive.

2. Observations are independent.

3. No category has an expected frequency of less than 5 (or when there are many categories, not more than 20% of the categories have an expected frequency of less than 5).

EXAMPLE 9.1   A Chi-Square Goodness of Fit Test

Two purple-flowered pea plants, both heterozygous for flower color, were crossed, resulting in 78 purple-flowered offspring and 22 white-flowered offspring. Does this outcome differ from a 3:1 ratio of purple-flowered to white-flowered offspring? ■

Color is controlled by a single pair of alleles, and purple is dominant over white. Because of this we expect a ratio of 3 purple-flowered offspring to 1 white-flowered offspring, based on a binomial probability (see chapter 5). Thus, we would expect 75 purple-flowered plants and 25 white-flowered plants (which is the null hypothesis). However, by chance alone we might expect that there would be some discrepancy between the expected results and what we actually obtained.

The question in a goodness of fit test is this: is this observed discrepancy between the observed frequencies and the expected frequencies too large to be attributed to chance alone? In other words, is the difference between the observed result and the expected result significant? The chi-square statistic is given by

$$\chi^2 = \Sigma \frac{(o - e)^2}{e} \tag{9.1}$$

The steps in its computation, shown in table 9.1, are as follows.

1. Subtract each expected value (column 2) from each observed value (column 1). The difference $(o - e)$ is shown in column 3.
2. Square the values of $(o - e)$, to obtain the squared differences, $(o - e)^2$, as shown in column 4.
3. Divide each squared difference by the expected value (e) for that category to obtain the value of $\frac{(o - e)^2}{e}$ for each category (column 5).
4. Sum the values obtained in column 5 to obtain chi-square.
5. The degrees of freedom for a chi-square goodness of fit test are the number of mutually exclusive groups minus one.

Table 9.1 Calculation of the Chi-Square Statistic

(1) observed	(2) expected	(3) $(o - e)$	(4) $(o - e)^2$	(5) $\dfrac{(o - e)^2}{e}$
78	75	3	9	0.12
22	25	−3	9	0.36

$$\chi^2 = \Sigma \frac{(o - e)^2}{e} = 0.48$$

We now consult table A.3, ''Critical Values of the Chi-Square Distribution.'' The top row of this table gives probabilities associated with values of chi-square, and the left column gives degrees of freedom. Our calculated value, 0.48 with one degree of freedom, is less than the critical value for alpha 0.05 and one degree of freedom. Therefore, we are unable to reject the null hypothesis. We conclude that the observed frequency does not differ from the expected frequency. Now let us look at a somewhat more complex situation.

EXAMPLE 9.2   A Chi-Square Goodness of Fit Test

Refer to the maple seedlings per quadrate example in chapter 4, which is reproduced here as table 9.2. We wish to know if the seedlings are nonrandomly distributed in the sampled habitat. ■

If the maple seedlings in the sampled area were randomly distributed, we would expect, on the basis of the Poisson distribution, to obtain the results given in the column headed ''Expected.'' These are the expected values and are derived from our expectation that the distribution will follow a Poisson distribution. This is the null hypothesis. If we reject the null hypothesis, we accept the alternative hypothesis that the seedlings are not randomly distributed. The observed results are shown in the column headed ''Observed.'' We compute chi-square as before, with one small difference. For the chi-square test to be valid, not more than 20% of the expected values should be less than 5 (assumption 3), and some of our expected values fall below this. We solve this problem simply by combining the last 3 values in both the observed and expected columns, which is an acceptable procedure provided that the meaning of the data is not lost in the process. Table 9.2 gives the results of the chi-square computations for this example.

Table 9.2 Expected and Observed Values of Maple Seedlings per Quadrate ($n = 100$, $\bar{x} = 1.41$) (Data from Table 4.4)

Seedlings/Quadrate	Observed		Expected		$\dfrac{(o - e)^2}{e}$
0	35		24.4		4.60
1	28		34.4		1.19
2	15		24.3		3.56
3	10		11.4		0.17
4	7		4.0		
5	5	12	1.1	5.36	8.22
6	0		0.26		——

$$\chi^2 = \Sigma \frac{(o - e)^2}{e} = 17.74$$

$$df = 4$$

There appear to be 4 degrees of freedom in this case (5 groups $-$ 1). However, when it is necessary to estimate one or more parameters in the population of interest, one degree of freedom must be deducted for each parameter estimated. Recall that in this case our expected values are based on our sample mean of 1.41 seedlings per quadrate. In other words, we are using an estimate of the population mean to obtain the expected values. Thus, the degrees of freedom are 3 rather than 4. Reference to table A.3 gives a critical value of χ^2 at alpha 0.05 and 3 degrees of freedom as 7.82. Since our calculated value is larger than this, we reject the null hypothesis and conclude that the maple seedlings are not randomly distributed in the sampled habitat because the observed distribution does not follow a Poisson distribution.

THE CHI-SQUARE TEST FOR ASSOCIATION

Tests for association are used to determine if 2 variables, both measured on a nominal scale, are related or associated in some way. It is helpful to think of these tests as tests for correlation between nominal variables. An example might help clarify this.

EXAMPLE 9.3   A Chi-Square Test for Association

In certain parts of West Africa where malaria is prevalent, there is a mutant form of hemoglobin called sickle-cell hemoglobin or hemoglobin S. Individuals who are homozygous for the hemoglobin S allele develop sickle-cell anemia, an often fatal disease. Individuals who are heterozygous exhibit some mild symptoms of anemia but have an abnormally high resistance to the malaria parasite. Individuals who are homozygous for normal hemoglobin are highly susceptible to malaria. The now infamous experiment that confirmed this is a good example of the relationship between 2 nominal variables—genotype and susceptibility to malaria—although the experiment itself would be regarded as inhumane and unethical by present standards. In this experiment 30 prison inmates, all volunteers, were selected. Fifteen of these individuals were heterozygous for hemoglobin S, and 15 were homozygous for normal hemoglobin. Otherwise, all 30 were from the same general population and were therefore genetically similar in other respects. All 30 were artificially infected with the malaria parasites! Of the 15 homozygous individuals, 13 contracted the disease, and 2 did not. Of the 15 heterozygous individuals, 1 contracted the disease, and the remaining 14 did not. Such data is customarily arrayed in the form of a matrix, sometimes called a contingency table, as shown in table 9.3.

Table 9.3 Association between the Hemoglobin S Allele and Resistance to Malaria

	Contracted Malaria	Did Not Contract Malaria	Totals
Heterozygotes	1	14	15
Homozygotes	13	2	15
Totals	14	16	30

The question asked in such an experiment is this: is there a relationship between the 2 variables? Remember, the 2 variables in this case are genotype (measured on a nominal scale) and susceptibility to malaria (also measured on a nominal scale). The null hypothesis is that there is no relationship (i.e., that the 2 variables are independent).

Assumptions of the Test

1. Data are frequencies.
2. Samples are *independent* (i.e., the same individual may not occur in more than one cell).
3. Not more than 20% of the cells may have an expected value of less than 5, and no cell may have an expected value of 0. This means that, for a 2 × 2 contingency table, all cells must have an expected value of 5 or greater.

Consider the experiment just outlined, which was conducted to determine if individuals who are heterozygous for the sickle-cell gene are more resistant to malaria than are homozygous normal individuals (example 9.3). The results are given again in table 9.4.

The expected value for each cell in a test for association is obtained by multiplying the row total by the column total for a cell, and then dividing the product by the grand total, or

$$\frac{\text{Row Total} \times \text{Column Total}}{\text{Grand Total}}$$

Table 9.4 Association between the Hemoglobin S Allele and Resistance to Malaria (Expected Values in Parentheses)

	Contracted Malaria	Did Not Contract Malaria	Totals
Heterozygotes	1 (7.00)	14 (8.00)	15
Homozygotes	13 (7.00)	2 (8.00)	15
Totals	14	16	30

As usual we compare the observed result with the result predicted by the null hypothesis, which is that there is no relationship between the heterozygous condition for this gene and resistance to malaria. We calculate a value for chi-square as before: by summing the values $\frac{(o - e)^2}{e}$ for each of the cells. Chi-square for this example is

$$\chi^2 = \frac{(1 - 7)^2}{7} + \frac{(14 - 8)^2}{8} + \frac{(13 - 7)^2}{7} + \frac{(2 - 8)^2}{8} = 19.2857$$

The degrees of freedom for a chi-square test for association are (rows $-$ 1) $\times$ (columns $-$ 1). In this case $(2 - 1) \times (2 - 1) = 1$. Consulting table A.3, we find that the critical value of chi-square at alpha 0.05 and one degree of freedom is 3.84. We therefore reject the null hypothesis and conclude that there is a relationship between heterozygosity for the sickle-cell gene and resistance to malaria.

The chi-square test for association is not limited to 2×2 contingency tables, and in fact, it may be expanded to as many rows and columns as necessary. Each row or each column would represent one mutually exclusive category into which an individual might fall. The procedure is exactly the same when there are more than 2 mutually exclusive categories, except that the degrees of freedom are greater than one. Example 9.4 illustrates this.

EXAMPLE 9.4   A Chi-Square Test for Association

An animal behaviorist wished to determine if the performance of 3 different olfactory behaviors, which bulls of a certain breed of cattle typically exhibit on approaching a female of their species, is related to the reproductive stage of the female. We will designate these behaviors as A, B, and C, and the reproductive stages of the females as conceptive or nonconceptive. We need not be concerned here with what these 3 behaviors are—only that they are mutually exclusive events. The data given in table 9.5 were obtained.   ■

Table 9.5 Frequencies of Three Olfactory Behaviors Directed to Cows by Bulls

Female	Behavior of Bull			
	A	B	C	Total
Conceptive	29 (29.78)	48 (56.64)	27 (17.58)	104
Nonconceptive	32 (31.22)	68 (59.36)	9 (18.42)	109
Total	61	116	36	213

Expected values, obtained by multiplying row totals by column totals and dividing by the grand total, are shown in parentheses. Chi-square is computed as before. In this case,

$$\chi^2 = \frac{(29 - 29.78)^2}{29.78} + \frac{(48 - 56.64)^2}{56.64} + \frac{(27 - 17.58)^2}{17.58}$$
$$+ \frac{(32 - 31.22)^2}{31.22} + \frac{(68 - 59.36)^2}{59.36} + \frac{(9 - 18.42)^2}{18.42} = 12.485$$

The degrees of freedom in this case are:

$$(r - 1) \times (c - 1) = (2 - 1) \times (3 - 1) = 2$$

As before, we consult table A.3, using 2 degrees of freedom, to determine if we may reject the null hypothesis that there is no association between the reproductive state of the female and the performance of these 3 behaviors by bulls.

THE FISHER EXACT PROBABILITY TEST

The Fisher exact probability test, like the chi-square test for association, is used to test for an association between 2 variables measured on a nominal scale. An important difference is that the requirement that no cell have an expected value of less than 5 is not applicable to the Fisher test, and accordingly, the test is very useful for small samples. The assumption of independence (i.e., that no individual may occupy more than one cell) must be satisfied.

EXAMPLE 9.5   The Fisher Exact Probability Test

An experiment was conducted to determine if neonatal garter snakes were more or less likely to exhibit an avoidance response to a threatening stimulus presented from above or from "snakes-eye level." One sample of 7 snakes was presented one at a time with an overhead stimulus, and another sample of 7 was presented with the same stimulus presented laterally. The investigator recorded whether the snakes responded by attempting to "escape" or failed to respond. (Data from R. Hampton and J. Gillingham)   ■

Two independent samples are involved here—snakes which were stimulated from above and snakes which were stimulated laterally—and 2 mutually exclusive categories—responded or did not respond. Measurement is nominal. To conduct the Fisher test, data of this type are arranged in a 2×2 contingency table, as in tables 9.6 and 9.7.

Table 9.6 Arrangement of Data for the Fisher Exact Probability Test

	Classification 1	Classification 2	Totals
Group I	A	B	A + B
Group II	C	D	C + D
Totals	A + C	B + D	A + B + C + D

The probability of observing this particular distribution if the null hypothesis of no association is true is given by

$$p = \frac{(A + B)! \, (C + D)! \, (A + C)! \, (B + D)!}{n! \, A! \, B! \, C! \, D!} \tag{9.2}$$

where $n = A + B + C + D$, and by convention $0! = 1$.

The data for the example are shown in table 9.7.

Table 9.7 Response of Neonatal Garter Snakes to Overhead and Lateral Stimuli

	Responded	No Response	Totals
Overhead Stimulus	6	1	7
Lateral Stimulus	1	6	7
Totals	7	7	14

The probability of this outcome under the null hypothesis is

$$p = \frac{7! \times 7! \times 7! \times 7!}{14! \times 6! \times 1! \times 1! \times 6!} = 0.01428$$

This is the probability of the observed distribution if H_0 is true. However, we are not interested in exactly this outcome, but of this outcome or of any more extreme outcomes with the same marginal totals. There is only one more extreme outcome in this case, which is:

	Responded	*No Response*	*Totals*
Overhead Stimulus	7	0	7
Lateral Stimulus	0	7	7
Totals	7	7	14

The probability for this case is

$$p = \frac{7! \times 7! \times 7! \times 7!}{14! \times 7! \times 0! \times 0! \times 7!} = 0.00029$$

Thus, the probability under H_0 of our observed distribution or of one even more extreme is $0.01428 + 0.00029 = 0.01457$. We may reject H_0 and conclude that neonatal garter snakes are more responsive to the overhead stimulus than to the eye-level stimulus.

The expected values in this example would be too small for the chi-square test for association. Therefore, the Fisher exact probability test was used. Of course, the Fisher test may be used when the expected values are large enough to permit use of the chi-square test for association. The only limitation on the use of the Fisher test, assuming that its assumptions are met, is the limit imposed by the fact that factorial numbers may become too large to deal with in a reasonable way.

CAUTION

An important assumption of all the tests for association we have considered in this chapter is that observations are independent. If the data do not meet this assumption, the probability of a type I error may actually be much higher than the test result indicates. Independent, in this case, means that no individual may occur in more than one cell of a contingency table. What exactly does this mean? Consider the example we discussed earlier in this chapter regarding the frequency with which bulls exhibited one of 3 behaviors in the presence of conceptive and nonconceptive cows. The total number of occurrences recorded in table 9.5 was 213. Thus, we would assume that 213 bulls were observed one time, each on approaching a cow in one of the 2 conditions of the test (note that it would not be necessary to have 213 cows). However, only 14 bulls were used in this experiment. Accordingly, each bull was observed an average of just over 15 times! This in itself is a serous violation of independence, but to make matters worse, we have no knowledge of how many times each bull was actually observed. Some may have been observed many times (meaning that they would make a large contribution to the results), while others might have been observed only a few times. This "pooling" (see chapter 1) causes the test to be very unreliable, and it is to be avoided without exception.

THE McNEMAR TEST FOR THE SIGNIFICANCE OF CHANGES

In some situations it is either not possible or not desirable to maintain strict statistical independence, as was previously pointed out in conjunction with the paired *t*-test and with repeated measures ANOVA. We might, for example, wish to expose the same set of individuals to 2 different treatments and measure their response, thus reducing the effect of variation between individuals that is not related to the treatments; or we might wish to measure a "before and after" treatment effect of some sort, measuring the response of each individual before the treatment and again after the treatment, in effect using each individual as its own control. In such cases, and provided that we have designed the experiment properly, it is possible to use the McNemar test. In this test our focus is on the number of individuals who change in response to the 2 treatments.

Assumptions of the Test

1. Data are measured on at least a nominal scale.
2. Each subject is measured twice: once under each of the 2 treatments.

EXAMPLE 9.6   The McNemar Test

Rattlesnakes kill their prey by striking and injecting venom. Sometimes they grasp the prey immediately and wait for it to die before ingesting it; at other times they release the prey after striking it, wait for it to die, and then grasp and ingest it. This decision seems to be related to the size of the prey. Presumably, a large prey item would be capable of inflicting injury to the snake while it is dying if the snake attempted to hold the prey in its mouth during this period, while a small prey item would be much less likely to inflict injury. This hypothesis predicts that large prey should be struck and released, while small prey items should be struck and held. (Such an experiment was conducted by R. K. Easter and M. A. Goodrick, but the data given below are fictitious.)

Fifteen rattlesnakes (*Crotalus atrox*) were each fed a mouse (small prey) and a rat (large prey). It was noted whether they struck and released or struck and held the prey. The results are shown in table 9.8.

Table 9.8   Data for Example 9.6

		Rat (Large Prey)			
		Released		Held	
Mouse	Released	3	(*a*)	0	(*b*)
(Small Prey)	Held	10	(*c*)	2	(*d*)

Those snakes that changed their response between the 2 treatments (large and small prey) are in cells *b* and *c*. Those that released small prey but held large prey occur in cell *b* (none did this). Those that held small prey but released large prey occur in cell *c* (10 did this). Animals in cells *a* and *d* either released both sizes (cell a) or held both sizes (cell d), which is to say that they did not change their response to the 2 treatments. In the McNemar test, we are interested only in the "changers."

The test statistic for the McNemar test is chi-square, which is computed as

$$\chi^2 = \frac{(c - b)^2}{(c + b)} \tag{9.3}$$

For the example,

$$\chi^2 = \frac{100}{10} = 10$$

There are $(r - 1) \times (c - 1) = 1$ degree of freedom. As before, if the calculated value of chi-square is greater than the tabular value with one degree of freedom, we may reject the null hypothesis that there is no change in individual responses to the 2 treatments.

When frequencies are sufficiently small such that $\frac{(c + b)}{2} < 5$, we may compute a binomial probability for the McNemar test. In this case $k = c + b$, $x =$ the smaller of the 2 frequencies in cells c or b, and $p = 0.5$.

EXAMPLE 9.7

Suppose that the outcome of our rattlesnake experiment described in example 9.6 had been as follows.

		Rat (Large Prey)	
		Released	Held
Mouse	Released	3 (a)	0 (b)
(Small Prey)	Held	9 (c)	3 (d)

The value for $\frac{(c + b)}{2}$ is now 4.5, and the use of chi-square is therefore inappropriate. We may use the binomial test by setting $k = c + b = 9$, $x = 0$ (the smaller of the 2 frequencies in cells b and c), and $p = 0.5$. Substituting these values in the binomial probability equation (chapter 4) gives

$$p(x) = \frac{k!}{x!\,(k - x)!}\, p^x \times q^{(k - x)} = 0.002$$

and we may reject the null hypothesis.

KEY TERMS

goodness of fit test   **test for association**

EXERCISES

(Exercises preceded by an asterisk are suitable for a computer solution.)

9.1   One hundred tweetie birds were given a choice of either striped sunflower seeds or black sunflower seeds. Seventy-five chose black seeds.

May we conclude that the population from which this sample was taken has a preference for black sunflower seeds over striped sunflower seeds?

9.2 Suppose that in the situation described in exercise 9.1, 48 tweetie birds had chosen black seeds, and 52 had chosen striped seeds. May we conclude that there is a preference for striped seeds?

9.3 In a genetic experiment involving flower color in a certain plant species, a ratio of 3 blue-flowered plants to 1 white-flowered plant was expected. The observed results were 35 blue-flowered plants and 14 white-flowered plants. Does the observed ratio differ significantly from the expected ratio?

9.4 Suppose that in exercise 9.3 a ratio of 61 blue-flowered plants to 22 white-flowered plants was observed. Does the observed ratio differ significantly from the expected ratio?

9.5 In snapdragons, red flower color is incompletely dominant. Homozygous dominant individuals are red, heterozygous individuals are pink, and homozygous recessive individuals are white. In a cross of 2 heterozygous individuals, a ratio of 1 red to 2 pink to 1 white is expected in the offspring. The results of such a cross were 10 red, 21 pink, and 9 white. Do the observed results differ significantly from a 1:2:1 ratio?

9.6 Suppose that the results in exercise 9.5 had been 8 red, 25 pink, and 7 white. Do the observed results differ significantly from a 1:2:1 ratio?

9.7 Based on our understanding of X and Y chromosomes, it is expected that female births equal male births in most mammalian species. In a sample of 60 individuals from a population, 28 were males, and 32 were females. May we conclude that the sex ratio in this population is something other than 1:1?

9.8 Suppose that in exercise 9.6 a ratio of 25 males to 35 females had been the observed sex ratio in the sample. Would this be reason to conclude that the population sex ratio is something other than 1:1?

9.9 We suspect that a certain strain of laboratory rats has a genetic tendency to make left turns in a "T" maze. Of 12 rats that were tested in such a maze, 8 chose to go into the left arm and 4 chose the right arm. Does this result support our suspicion about a left-turning tendency?

*9.10 Using the chi-square goodness of fit test and the data from table B.2, determine if the total length of female mosquito fish is approximately normally distributed.

*9.11 Using the chi-square goodness of fit test and the data from table B.2, determine if the total length of male mosquito fish is approximately normally distributed.

*9.12 Using the chi-square goodness of fit test and the data from table B.1, determine if bluegill standard length is approximately normally distributed.

*9.13 Using the chi-square goodness of fit test and the data from table B.3, determine if the resting pulse rate of human females is approximately normally distributed.

9.14 It is suspected that male offspring or female offspring tend to "run in families" (i.e., some families seem to produce mostly boys, others mostly girls). To test this idea, 185 litters of bush hogs, each containing 6 hoglets, were surveyed. The number of males and the number of females in each litter was determined, with the following results.

Males	Females	Number of Litters Observed
0	6	10
1	5	20
2	4	36
3	3	47
4	2	32
5	1	28
6	1	12

Do the observations support the suspicion? (See examples 4.1 and 4.2 in chapter 4 for a refresher on how to determine the expected values in this situation.)

9.15 In 102 tosses of 4 coins, the following results were obtained.

Heads	Tails	Observed Frequency
4	0	8
3	1	23
2	2	40
1	3	27
0	4	4

Does this outcome differ significantly from what would be predicted by chance alone?

9.16 In 120 rolls of 5 dice, the following results were obtained.

Number of Sixes	Observed Frequency
5	6
4	8
3	12
2	20
1	39
0	35

Assuming that the dice are "fair," is it likely that this outcome would occur by chance alone? (Or more to the point, would you care to gamble with the owner of these dice?)

9.17 Forty-seven groups of common suckers, each consisting of 3 individuals, were surveyed during their spawning season. The sex ratio in the population may be assumed to be 1:1. The number of males and females in each group of 3 were as follows.

Males	Females	Frequency
3	0	7
2	1	35
1	2	3
0	3	2

Is it likely that the number of males and females in groups of 3 individuals are due to chance alone?

9.18 Refer to example 4.4 concerning the number of maple seedlings per quadrate in a random sample of 100 quadrates. Using the sample mean as the best estimate of the parametric mean, determine if the observed results follow Poisson distribution. Interpret your results biologically.

9.19 Refer to exercise 2.3 concerning the distribution of ant lion pits. Using the sample mean as the best estimate of the parametric mean, determine if the distribution of pits follows a Poisson distribution. Interpret your results biologically.

9.20 Refer to exercise 2.4 and your calculations from exercise 4.28 concerning the number of chironomid larvae found in pitcher plant leaves. Using the sample mean as the best estimate of the population mean, determine if this variable (larvae/leaf) fits a Poisson distribution.

9.21 It is suspected that female water snakes that forage in Lake Michigan migrate to inland ponds in the fall to deliver their young. If this is correct, one might expect that females would be much more likely to migrate at that time than would males. The following data were collected.

	Migrators	Nonmigrators
Females	25	2
Males	4	30

Data from C. Meyers

Is there an association between sex and migration?

9.22 White-throated sparrows occur in 2 distinct color morphs, referred to as brown and white. It was suspected that females select mates of the opposite morph (i.e., white females select brown males and vice versa). This phenomenon is known as negative assortative mating. In 30 mated pairs, the color combinations were as follows.

		Males	
		White	Brown
Females	White	7	23
	Brown	14	5

Data from D. Tuzzalino

Do the results support the assumption that negative assortative mating occurs in this species?

9.23 In territorial pairs of convict cichlids (*Chiclasoma nigrofasciatum*), either member of the resident pair is likely to attack a conspecific intruder into the territory. It is suspected that the resident male is more likely to attack an intruding male, and that the resident female is more likely to attack an intruding female. In 35 aggressive interactions, each involving a different resident pair, the following results were obtained.

		Intruder	
		Male	Female
Resident	Male	12	5
	Female	3	15

9.24 The presence of a certain gene in samples of juniper pythons from 2 geographically isolated populations was measured. The data following are the number of snakes that had and that did not have the gene in each of the populations. Is there an association between location and the frequency of this gene in the population?

	Location A	Location B
Gene Present	20	5
Gene Absent	6	30

*9.25   Using the data from table B.3 (see appendix B), determine if male university students are more or less likely to smoke than are female university students (i.e., determine if there is an association between smoking and sex).

*9.26   Using the data from table B.3, determine if male university students are more or less likely to participate in a varsity sport than are female university students (i.e., determine if there is an association between sex and participation in a varsity sport).

*9.27   Using the data from table B.3, determine if male university students are more or less likely to do aerobic exercises on a regular basis than are female university students (i.e., determine if there is an association between sex and aerobic exercising).

*9.28   Using the data from table B.3, determine if male university students are more or less likely to participate in weight training than are female university students (i.e., determine if there is an association between sex and weight training).

9.29   The frequency of 3 food items (small snails, cladocerians, and mosquito larvae) in the stomach contents of male and female mosquito fish was determined. Do males and females differ with respect to food items utilized?

		Food Item		
		Snail	Cladocerian	Mosquito Larvae
Sex	Males	50	23	15
	Females	10	14	62

9.30   Suppose that the outcome of exercise 9.22 had been as follows.

		Males	
		White	Brown
Females	White	1	6
	Brown	5	2

Determine if the null hypothesis of no association may be rejected.

9.31   Using the data from exercise 9.21, conduct the Fisher exact probability test to determine if the null hypothesis of no association may be rejected.

9.32   Using the data from exercise 9.24, conduct the Fisher exact probability test to determine if the null hypothesis of no association may be rejected.

9.33   Redesign example 9.5 as a repeated-measures experiment in such a way that the McNemar test could be used.

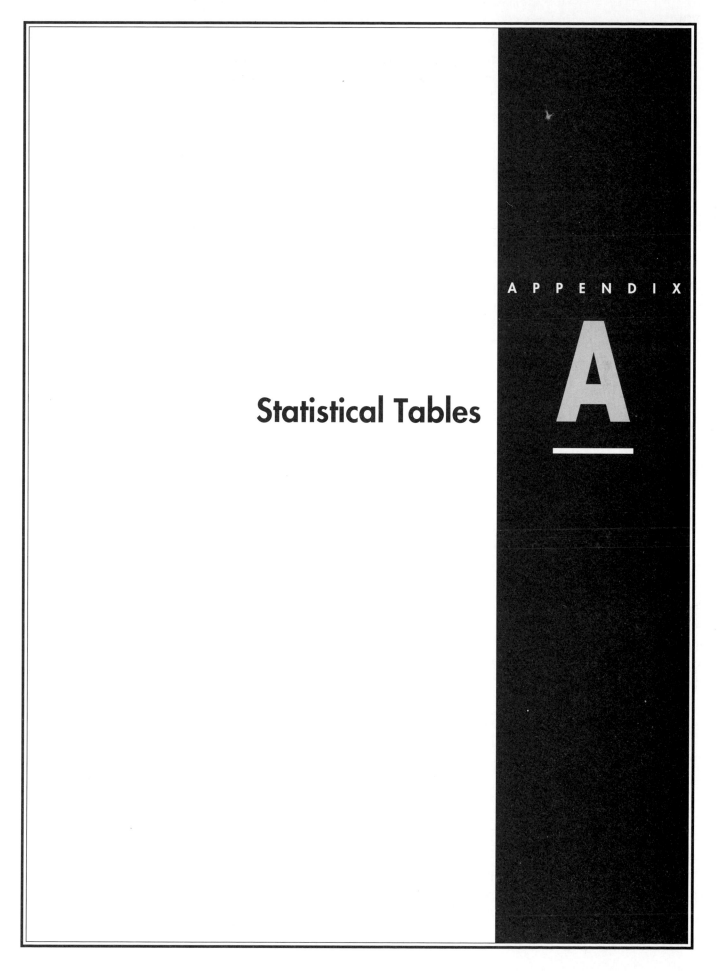

Statistical Tables

TABLE A.1   AREAS OF THE NORMAL DISTRIBUTION

z	0.00	0.01	0.02	0.03	0.04	0.05	0.06	0.07	0.08	0.09
0.0	0.0000	0.0040	0.0080	0.0120	0.0160	0.0199	0.0239	0.0279	0.0319	0.0359
0.1	0.0398	0.0438	0.0478	0.0517	0.0557	0.0596	0.0636	0.0675	0.0714	0.0754
0.2	0.0793	0.0832	0.0871	0.0910	0.0948	0.0987	0.1026	0.1064	0.1103	0.1141
0.3	0.1179	0.1217	0.1255	0.1293	0.1331	0.1368	0.1406	0.1443	0.1480	0.1517
0.4	0.1554	0.1591	0.1628	0.1664	0.1700	0.1736	0.1772	0.1808	0.1844	0.1879
0.5	0.1915	0.1950	0.1985	0.2019	0.2054	0.2088	0.2123	0.2157	0.2190	0.2224
0.6	0.2258	0.2291	0.2324	0.2357	0.2389	0.2422	0.2454	0.2486	0.2518	0.2549
0.7	0.2580	0.2612	0.2642	0.2673	0.2704	0.2734	0.2764	0.2794	0.2823	0.2852
0.8	0.2881	0.2910	0.2939	0.2967	0.2996	0.3023	0.3051	0.3078	0.3106	0.3133
0.9	0.3159	0.3186	0.3212	0.3238	0.3264	0.3289	0.3315	0.3340	0.3365	0.3389
1.0	0.3413	0.3438	0.3461	0.3485	0.3508	0.3531	0.3554	0.3577	0.3599	0.3621
1.1	0.3643	0.3665	0.3686	0.3708	0.3729	0.3749	0.3770	0.3790	0.3810	0.3830
1.2	0.3849	0.3869	0.3888	0.3907	0.3925	0.3944	0.3962	0.3980	0.3997	0.4015
1.3	0.4032	0.4049	0.4066	0.4082	0.4099	0.4115	0.4131	0.4147	0.4162	0.4177
1.4	0.4192	0.4207	0.4222	0.4236	0.4251	0.4265	0.4279	0.4292	0.4306	0.4319
1.5	0.4332	0.4345	0.4357	0.4370	0.4382	0.4394	0.4406	0.4418	0.4429	0.4441
1.6	0.4452	0.4463	0.4474	0.4484	0.4495	0.4505	0.4515	0.4525	0.4535	0.4545
1.7	0.4554	0.4564	0.4573	0.4582	0.4591	0.4599	0.4608	0.4616	0.4625	0.4633
1.8	0.4641	0.4649	0.4656	0.4664	0.4671	0.4678	0.4686	0.4693	0.4699	0.4706
1.9	0.4713	0.4719	0.4726	0.4732	0.4738	0.4744	0.4750	0.4756	0.4761	0.4767
2.0	0.4772	0.4778	0.4783	0.4788	0.4793	0.4798	0.4803	0.4808	0.4812	0.4817
2.1	0.4821	0.4826	0.4830	0.4834	0.4838	0.4842	0.4846	0.4850	0.4854	0.4857
2.2	0.4861	0.4864	0.4868	0.4871	0.4875	0.4878	0.4881	0.4884	0.4887	0.4890
2.3	0.4893	0.4896	0.4898	0.4901	0.4904	0.4906	0.4909	0.4911	0.4913	0.4916
2.4	0.4918	0.4920	0.4922	0.4925	0.4927	0.4929	0.4931	0.4932	0.4934	0.4936
2.5	0.4938	0.4940	0.4941	0.4943	0.4945	0.4946	0.4948	0.4949	0.4951	0.4952
2.6	0.4953	0.4955	0.4956	0.4957	0.4959	0.4960	0.4961	0.4962	0.4963	0.4964
2.7	0.4965	0.4966	0.4967	0.4968	0.4969	0.4970	0.4971	0.4972	0.4973	0.4974
2.8	0.4974	0.4975	0.4976	0.4977	0.4977	0.4978	0.4979	0.4979	0.4980	0.4981
2.9	0.4981	0.4982	0.4982	0.4983	0.4984	0.4984	0.4985	0.4985	0.4986	0.4986
3.0	0.4987	0.4987	0.4987	0.4988	0.4988	0.4989	0.4989	0.4989	0.4990	0.4990
3.1	0.4990	0.4991	0.4991	0.4991	0.4992	0.4992	0.4992	0.4992	0.4993	0.4993
3.2	0.4993	0.4993	0.4994	0.4994	0.4994	0.4994	0.4994	0.4995	0.4995	0.4995
3.3	0.4995	0.4995	0.4995	0.4996	0.4996	0.4996	0.4996	0.4996	0.4996	0.4997
3.4	0.4997	0.4997	0.4997	0.4997	0.4997	0.4997	0.4997	0.4997	0.4997	0.4998
3.5	0.4998	0.4998	0.4998	0.4998	0.4998	0.4998	0.4998	0.4998	0.4998	0.4998
3.6	0.4998	0.4998	0.4999	0.4999	0.4999	0.4999	0.4999	0.4999	0.4999	0.4999
3.7	0.4999	0.4999	0.4999	0.4999	0.4999	0.4999	0.4999	0.4999	0.4999	0.4999
3.8	0.4999	0.4999	0.4999	0.4999	0.4999	0.4999	0.4999	0.4999	0.4999	0.4999
3.9	0.49995	0.49995	0.49996	0.49996	0.49996	0.49996	0.49996	0.49996	0.49997	0.49997

TABLE A.2   CRITICAL VALUES OF THE t DISTRIBUTION

df	\(\alpha\) (Two-Tailed)					
	0.1	**0.05**	**0.02**	**0.01**	**0.001**	**0.0001**
1	6.314	12.706	31.821	63.657	636.619	6,366.198
2	2.920	4.303	6.695	9.925	31.598	99.992
3	2.353	3.182	4.541	5.841	12.924	28.000
4	2.132	2.776	3.747	4.604	8.610	15.544
5	2.015	2.571	3.365	4.032	6.869	11.178
6	1.943	2.447	3.143	3.707	5.959	9.082
7	1.895	2.365	2.998	3.499	5.408	7.885
8	1.860	2.306	2.896	3.355	5.041	7.120
9	1.833	2.262	2.821	3.250	4.781	6.594
10	1.812	2.228	2.764	3.169	4.587	6.211
11	1.796	2.201	2.718	3.106	4.437	5.921
12	1.782	2.179	2.681	3.055	4.318	5.694
13	1.771	2.160	2.650	3.012	4.221	5.513
14	1.761	2.145	2.624	2.977	4.140	5.363
15	1.753	2.131	2.602	2.947	4.073	5.239
16	1.746	2.120	2.583	2.921	4.015	5.134
17	1.740	2.110	2.567	2.898	3.965	5.044
18	1.734	2.101	2.552	2.878	3.922	4.966
19	1.729	2.093	2.539	2.861	3.883	4.897
20	1.725	2.086	2.528	2.845	3.850	4.837
21	1.721	2.080	2.518	2.831	3.819	4.784
22	1.717	2.074	2.508	2.819	3.792	4.736
23	1.714	2.069	2.500	2.807	3.767	4.693
24	1.711	2.064	2.492	2.797	3.745	4.654
25	1.708	2.060	2.485	2.787	3.725	4.619
26	1.706	2.056	2.479	2.779	3.707	4.587
27	1.703	2.052	2.473	2.771	3.690	4.558
28	1.701	2.048	2.467	2.763	3.674	4.530
29	1.699	2.045	2.462	2.756	3.659	4.506
30	1.697	2.042	2.457	2.750	3.646	4.482
40	1.684	2.021	2.423	2.704	3.551	4.321
60	1.671	2.000	2.390	2.660	3.460	4.169
100	1.660	1.984	2.364	2.626	3.390	4.053

TABLE A.3 CRITICAL VALUES OF THE CHI-SQUARE DISTRIBUTION

df	0.05	0.02	α 0.01	0.001	0.0001
1	3.84	5.41	6.63	10.83	15.14
2	5.99	7.82	9.21	13.82	18.42
3	7.81	9.84	11.34	16.27	21.11
4	9.49	11.67	13.28	18.47	23.51
5	11.07	13.39	15.09	20.51	25.74
6	12.59	15.03	16.81	22.46	27.86
7	14.07	16.62	18.48	24.32	29.88
8	15.51	18.17	20.09	26.12	31.83
9	16.92	19.68	21.67	27.88	33.72
10	18.31	21.16	23.21	29.59	35.56
11	19.68	22.62	24.72	31.26	37.37
12	21.03	24.05	26.22	32.91	39.13
13	22.36	25.47	27.69	34.53	40.87
14	23.68	26.87	29.14	36.12	42.58
15	25.00	28.26	30.58	37.70	44.26
16	26.30	29.63	32.00	39.25	45.92
17	27.59	31.00	33.41	40.79	47.57
18	28.87	32.35	34.81	42.31	49.19
19	30.14	33.69	36.19	43.82	50.80
20	31.41	35.02	37.57	45.31	52.39
21	32.67	36.34	38.93	46.80	53.96
22	33.92	37.66	40.29	48.27	55.52
23	35.17	38.97	41.64	49.73	57.08
24	36.42	40.27	42.98	51.18	58.61
25	37.65	41.57	44.31	52.62	60.14
26	38.89	42.86	45.64	54.05	61.66
27	40.11	44.14	46.96	55.48	63.16
28	41.34	45.42	48.28	56.89	64.66
29	42.56	46.69	49.59	58.30	66.15
30	43.77	47.96	50.89	59.70	67.63

TABLE A.4   **CRITICAL VALUES OF *U* FOR THE MANN-WHITNEY TEST ($\alpha = 0.05$, TWO-TAILED; n_1 AND n_2 ARE THE TWO SAMPLE SIZES)**

								n_1									
5	6	7	8	9	10	11	12	13	14	15	16	17	18	19	20	n_2
23	27	30	34	38	42	46	49	53	57	61	65	68	72	76	80	5
	31	36	40	44	49	53	58	62	67	71	75	80	84	89	93	6
		41	46	51	56	61	66	71	76	81	86	91	96	101	106	7
			51	57	63	69	74	80	86	91	97	102	108	114	119	8
				64	70	76	82	89	95	101	107	114	120	126	132	9
					77	84	91	97	104	111	118	125	132	138	145	10
						91	99	106	114	121	129	136	143	151	158	11
							107	115	123	131	139	147	155	163	171	12
								124	132	141	149	158	167	175	184	13
									141	151	160	169	178	188	197	14
										161	170	180	190	200	210	15
											181	191	202	212	222	16
												202	213	224	235	17
													225	236	248	18
														248	261	19
															273	20

TABLE A.5   **CRITICAL VALUES OF *T* FOR THE WILCOXON TEST (TWO-TAILED PROBABILITIES; *n* IS THE NUMBER OF MATCHED PAIRS)**

	α	
n	0.05	0.01
6	0	–
7	2	–
8	4	0
9	6	2
10	8	3
11	11	5
12	14	7
13	17	10
14	21	13
15	25	16
16	30	20
17	35	23
18	40	28
19	46	32
20	52	38
21	59	43
22	66	49
23	73	55
24	81	61
25	89	68

TABLE A.6   CRITICAL VALUES OF THE _F_ DISTRIBUTION ($\alpha = 0.05$; df_1 = TREATMENT DEGREES OF FREEDOM, df_2 = ERROR DEGREES OF FREEDOM)

df_2	df_1 1	2	3	4	5	6	7	8	9	10	11	12
2	18.5	19.0	19.2	19.3	19.4	19.4	19.4	19.4	19.4	19.4	19.4	19.4
3	10.1	9.55	9.28	9.12	9.01	8.94	8.89	8.85	8.81	8.79	8.76	8.74
4	7.71	6.94	6.59	6.39	6.26	6.16	6.09	6.04	6.00	5.96	5.93	5.91
5	6.61	5.79	5.41	5.19	5.05	4.95	4.88	4.82	4.77	4.74	4.71	4.68
6	5.99	5.14	4.76	4.53	4.39	4.28	4.21	4.15	4.10	4.06	4.03	4.00
7	5.59	4.74	4.35	4.12	3.97	3.87	3.77	3.73	3.68	3.64	3.60	3.57
8	5.32	4.46	4.07	3.84	3.69	3.58	3.50	3.44	3.39	3.35	3.31	3.28
9	5.12	4.26	3.86	3.63	3.48	3.37	3.29	3.23	3.18	3.14	3.10	3.07
10	4.96	4.10	3.71	3.48	3.33	3.22	3.14	3.07	3.02	2.98	2.94	2.91
11	4.84	3.98	3.59	3.36	3.20	3.09	3.01	2.95	2.90	2.85	2.82	2.79
12	4.75	3.89	3.49	3.26	3.11	3.00	2.91	2.85	2.80	2.75	2.72	2.69
15	4.54	3.68	3.29	3.06	2.90	2.79	2.71	2.64	2.59	2.54	2.51	2.48
20	4.35	3.49	3.10	2.87	2.71	2.60	2.51	2.45	2.39	2.35	2.31	2.28
25	4.24	3.39	2.99	2.76	2.60	2.49	2.40	2.34	2.28	2.24	2.21	2.16
30	4.17	3.32	2.92	2.69	2.53	2.42	2.33	2.27	2.21	2.16	2.13	2.09
40	4.08	3.23	2.84	2.61	2.45	2.34	2.25	2.18	2.12	2.08	2.04	2.04
60	4.00	3.15	2.76	2.53	2.37	2.25	2.17	2.10	2.04	1.99	1.95	1.92
120	3.92	3.07	2.68	2.45	2.29	2.17	2.09	2.02	1.96	1.91	1.87	1.83

TABLE A.7   CRITICAL VALUES OF q (STUDENTIZED t) FOR THE TUKEY TEST ($\alpha = 0.05$)

Error df	Number of Groups (Treatments)								
	2	**3**	**4**	**5**	**6**	**7**	**8**	**9**	**10**
1	17.97	26.98	32.82	37.08	40.41	43.12	45.40	47.36	49.07
2	6.08	8.33	9.80	10.88	11.74	12.44	13.03	13.54	13.99
3	4.50	5.91	6.82	7.50	8.04	8.48	8.85	9.18	9.46
4	3.93	5.04	5.76	6.29	6.71	7.05	7.35	7.60	7.83
5	3.64	4.60	5.22	5.67	6.03	6.33	6.58	6.80	6.99
6	3.46	4.34	4.90	5.30	5.63	5.90	6.12	6.32	6.49
7	3.34	4.16	4.68	5.06	5.36	5.61	5.82	6.00	6.16
8	3.26	4.04	4.53	4.89	5.17	5.40	5.60	5.77	5.92
9	3.20	3.95	4.41	4.76	5.02	5.24	5.43	5.59	5.74
10	3.15	3.88	4.33	4.65	4.91	5.12	5.30	5.46	5.60
11	3.11	3.82	4.26	4.57	4.82	5.03	5.20	5.35	5.49
12	3.08	3.77	4.20	4.51	4.75	4.95	5.12	5.27	5.39
13	3.06	3.73	4.15	4.45	4.69	4.88	5.05	5.19	5.32
14	3.03	3.70	4.11	4.41	4.64	4.83	4.99	5.13	5.25
15	3.01	3.67	4.08	4.37	4.59	4.78	4.94	5.08	5.20
16	3.00	3.65	4.05	4.33	4.56	4.74	4.90	5.03	5.15
17	2.98	3.63	4.02	4.30	4.52	4.70	4.86	4.99	5.11
18	2.97	3.61	4.00	4.28	4.49	4.67	4.82	4.96	5.07
19	2.96	3.59	3.98	4.25	4.47	4.65	4.79	4.92	5.04
20	2.95	3.58	3.96	4.23	4.45	4.62	4.77	4.90	5.01
24	2.92	3.53	3.90	4.17	4.37	4.54	4.68	4.81	4.92
30	2.89	3.49	3.85	4.10	4.30	4.46	4.60	4.72	4.82
40	2.86	3.44	3.79	4.04	4.23	4.39	4.52	4.63	4.73
60	2.83	3.40	3.74	3.98	4.16	4.31	4.44	4.55	4.65
120	2.80	3.36	3.68	3.92	4.10	4.24	4.36	4.47	4.56
χ	2.77	3.31	3.63	3.86	4.03	4.17	4.29	4.39	4.47

TABLE A.8   CRITICAL VALUES OF THE PEARSON CORRELATION COEFFICIENT (r) ($\alpha = 0.05$)*

df	r	df	r
1	0.997	21	0.413
2	0.950	22	0.404
3	0.878	23	0.396
4	0.811	24	0.388
5	0.754	25	0.381
6	0.707	26	0.374
7	0.666	27	0.367
8	0.632	28	0.361
9	0.602	29	0.355
10	0.576	30	0.349
11	0.553	35	0.325
12	0.532	40	0.304
13	0.514	45	0.288
14	0.497	50	0.273
15	0.482	60	0.250
16	0.468	70	0.232
17	0.456	80	0.217
18	0.444	90	0.205
19	0.433	100	0.195
20	0.423	120	0.174

*For values not in the table, test for significance by the t-test.

TABLE A.9   CRITICAL VALUES OF THE SPEARMAN RANK CORRELATION COEFFICIENT ($\alpha = 0.05$)*

n	r_s
4	1.000
5	0.900
6	0.829
7	0.714
8	0.643
9	0.600
10	0.564
12	0.506
14	0.456
16	0.425
18	0.399
20	0.377

*For sample sizes not tabulated, test for significance using the t-test.

TABLE A.10   TABLE OF RANDOM NUMBERS

874335	218040	632420	240295	301131	152740	433058	274170
142131	051859	719342	714391	174251	147150	108520	771712
577728	460401	847722	767239	201744	006565	204589	960553
080052	246887	107893	627841	196599	792021	038162	390011
501153	355165	168311	790826	174928	955178	754258	125025
146207	369709	775557	516449	855970	838321	826020	246163
273515	015616	254341	330587	162088	174360	554720	349616
594504	658609	007492	524747	718771	586831	569750	047201
773722	805035	015969	656055	354632	089893	328631	466358
928848	601866	338853	047266	601409	588331	617007	750155
130680	336701	613351	286758	193966	377556	048648	557283
903145	937763	554796	728537	570290	643603	565449	562057
723294	473898	456644	992231	371495	963132	937428	954420
521302	654580	690478	463092	941820	803428	262731	939938
180471	329905	206005	792002	828627	022402	467626	239803
037226	990598	031055	395463	282404	368588	806509	590830
381118	268005	771588	955604	756766	981147	361899	245461
954822	434100	111684	920179	408451	889864	544440	471762
454139	901479	313550	002567	597321	515148	592903	053426
027996	723365	717520	681773	386364	168036	074181	789768
778443	093607	242049	702424	041696	550187	383294	995730
260656	846676	883719	574775	532552	253887	243386	001878
982935	957671	217239	074705	031298	262045	205728	654403
906706	042314	895439	743718	413420	448197	149714	815122
946521	856953	149277	388942	757533	076503	782862	861477
470054	798560	287835	583131	845375	301748	140819	186534
798107	404733	198320	164665	661808	669342	087352	698984
704605	853694	846064	737547	894822	615321	814358	323143
916600	464292	774523	171407	435529	966344	341855	498953
614267	196000	605281	101497	878168	439697	017987	681981
930906	148913	538043	428698	020102	143290	019025	843417
452944	063756	850643	819512	361819	075658	849363	970079
719931	821876	399037	206069	606933	625961	841521	564408
724544	945246	117307	286123	162181	073984	656142	144469
412582	096463	517660	023052	637428	090138	781997	743955
182972	578750	190428	145861	345662	235457	035980	412182
387765	835955	304068	649179	802995	461602	063111	714091
832135	952549	105163	293258	228666	610859	836534	230248
274385	153632	418418	103979	045038	916136	157518	056846
925940	304925	146667	872845	377600	500970	155459	305700

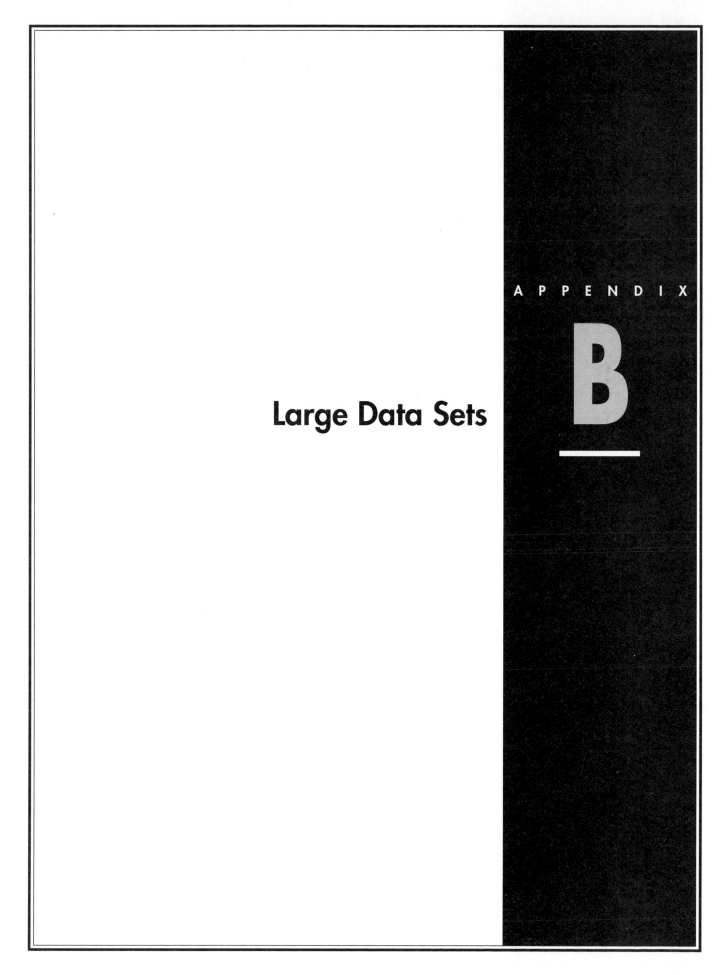

APPENDIX

B

Large Data Sets

TABLE B.1   LENGTH (IN MILLIMETERS) OF 888 BLUEGILL SUNFISH

Record Number	Length	Record Number	Length	Record Number	Length	Record Number	Length
1	151	51	50	101	156	151	160
2	182	52	54	102	140	152	162
3	182	53	55	103	159	153	157
4	162	54	50	104	80	154	155
5	177	55	55	105	155	155	146
6	166	56	54	106	78	156	155
7	197	57	80	107	158	157	143
8	144	58	80	108	67	158	154
9	174	59	92	109	57	159	157
10	172	60	54	110	165	160	141
11	174	61	76	111	81	161	150
12	160	62	70	112	155	162	142
13	53	63	71	113	141	163	139
14	50	64	54	114	180	164	137
15	52	65	72	115	145	165	72
16	64	66	50	116	145	166	66
17	53	67	156	117	150	167	146
18	53	68	56	118	76	168	130
19	52	69	68	119	145	169	126
20	51	70	52	120	135	170	85
21	55	71	54	121	82	171	179
22	56	72	56	122	88	172	80
23	51	73	54	123	105	173	75
24	63	74	125	124	122	174	138
25	57	75	51	125	75	175	75
26	56	76	51	126	74	176	70
27	53	77	54	127	84	177	72
28	51	78	52	128	77	178	87
29	59	79	56	129	76	179	103
30	51	80	56	130	72	180	163
31	57	81	54	131	180	181	80
32	51	82	55	132	75	182	135
33	131	83	55	133	152	183	157
34	85	84	52	134	87	184	150
35	80	85	56	135	161	185	129
36	55	86	50	136	170	186	84
37	50	87	51	137	156	187	89
38	84	88	46	138	150	188	72
39	52	89	170	139	122	189	147
40	53	90	74	140	140	190	153
41	53	91	64	141	77	191	84
42	75	92	153	142	85	192	150
43	56	93	86	143	80	193	140
44	68	94	52	144	133	194	146
45	60	95	72	145	145	195	138
46	54	96	172	146	190	196	154
47	51	97	146	147	165	197	137
48	59	98	127	148	176	198	189
49	75	99	65	149	170	199	165
50	52	100	93	150	145	200	142

TABLE B.1   Continued

Record Number	Length	Record Number	Length	Record Number	Length	Record Number	Length
201	140	251	81	301	74	351	151
202	141	252	138	302	75	352	170
203	160	253	75	303	68	353	168
204	125	254	125	304	135	354	137
205	156	255	173	305	142	355	204
206	145	256	175	306	75	356	154
207	159	257	220	307	140	357	179
208	147	258	172	308	131	358	191
209	155	259	132	309	88	359	149
210	178	260	163	310	100	360	171
211	80	261	139	311	155	361	162
212	195	262	142	312	171	362	185
213	71	263	180	313	169	363	175
214	82	264	152	314	83	364	180
215	94	265	157	315	153	365	164
216	80	266	165	316	84	366	205
217	70	267	147	317	84	367	168
218	74	268	154	318	74	368	178
219	81	269	167	319	80	369	139
220	76	270	167	320	74	370	158
221	175	271	155	321	76	371	134
222	110	272	159	322	73	372	179
223	80	273	149	323	73	373	179
224	77	274	172	324	158	374	127
225	105	275	202	325	156	375	149
226	86	276	155	326	160	376	149
227	67	277	149	327	80	377	148
228	70	278	144	328	75	378	152
229	149	279	162	329	152	379	77
230	158	280	165	330	70	380	141
231	139	281	156	331	75	381	154
232	128	282	140	332	76	382	112
233	105	283	154	333	164	383	145
234	68	284	158	334	114	384	125
235	144	285	182	335	84	385	142
236	119	286	135	336	80	386	74
237	117	287	163	337	78	387	100
238	115	288	155	338	76	388	142
239	120	289	173	339	144	389	139
240	75	290	83	340	181	390	140
241	174	291	75	341	175	391	142
242	133	292	75	342	201	392	140
243	143	293	76	343	200	393	118
244	145	294	84	344	171	394	134
245	177	295	86	345	201	395	138
246	79	296	70	346	195	396	131
247	86	297	81	347	195	397	144
248	87	298	78	348	194	398	142
249	87	299	146	349	191	399	140
250	156	300	115	350	180	400	132

(*Continued on p. 206*)

TABLE B.1   Continued

Record Number	Length	Record Number	Length	Record Number	Length	Record Number	Length
401	133	451	168	501	131	551	166
402	206	452	154	502	164	552	136
403	77	453	143	503	153	553	139
404	147	454	159	504	135	554	150
405	139	455	177	505	154	555	143
406	137	456	170	506	74	556	156
407	133	457	145	507	140	557	145
408	162	458	144	508	184	558	140
409	153	459	138	509	85	559	69
410	160	460	154	510	70	560	65
411	187	461	125	511	75	561	134
412	164	462	174	512	80	562	179
413	166	463	169	513	81	563	159
414	154	464	170	514	85	564	176
415	174	465	156	515	75	565	157
416	115	466	166	516	84	566	154
417	157	467	141	517	68	567	160
418	161	468	171	518	80	568	74
419	166	469	155	519	161	569	160
420	136	470	157	520	73	570	72
421	185	471	119	521	93	571	134
422	143	472	177	522	158	572	152
423	152	473	152	523	170	573	147
424	120	474	150	524	154	574	144
425	146	475	149	525	155	575	125
426	177	476	160	526	146	576	135
427	155	477	152	527	160	577	136
428	179	478	147	528	180	578	162
429	156	479	148	529	140	579	160
430	157	480	160	530	150	580	137
431	100	481	145	531	148	581	155
432	101	482	114	532	160	582	139
433	195	483	162	533	126	583	177
434	73	484	160	534	146	584	162
435	138	485	153	535	144	585	130
436	77	486	144	536	168	586	136
437	86	487	184	537	77	587	132
438	202	488	166	538	153	588	149
439	179	489	129	539	113	589	156
440	162	490	164	540	189	590	142
441	189	491	149	541	150	591	136
442	161	492	157	542	147	592	149
443	169	493	188	543	152	593	138
444	149	494	154	544	149	594	130
445	170	495	166	545	147	595	129
446	170	496	132	546	147	596	140
447	155	497	180	547	119	597	170
448	212	498	124	548	123	598	115
449	158	499	145	549	179	599	155
450	166	500	140	550	160	600	150

TABLE B.1   Continued

Record Number	Length	Record Number	Length	Record Number	Length	Record Number	Length
601	146	651	76	701	159	751	82
602	136	652	82	702	138	752	142
603	136	653	109	703	158	753	136
604	173	654	92	704	153	754	135
605	153	655	75	705	89	755	149
606	138	656	73	706	88	756	125
607	147	657	70	707	147	757	136
608	161	658	81	708	154	758	69
609	133	659	82	709	56	759	73
610	84	660	120	710	76	760	73
611	159	661	115	711	161	761	138
612	134	662	72	712	152	762	82
613	72	663	83	713	47	763	131
614	68	664	83	714	140	764	136
615	72	665	75	715	152	765	103
616	95	666	75	716	98	766	83
617	91	667	78	717	80	767	187
618	72	668	85	718	128	768	70
619	78	669	79	719	158	769	167
620	78	670	81	720	136	770	172
621	89	671	83	721	155	771	145
622	79	672	69	722	160	772	156
623	69	673	78	723	166	773	149
624	78	674	76	724	149	774	150
625	83	675	75	725	129	775	157
626	73	676	70	726	153	776	148
627	65	677	78	727	144	777	192
628	104	678	86	728	145	778	131
629	79	679	77	729	141	779	158
630	92	680	77	730	155	780	161
631	80	681	75	731	135	781	147
632	65	682	135	732	143	782	144
633	129	683	75	733	153	783	154
634	65	684	72	734	116	784	169
635	80	685	79	735	173	785	144
636	74	686	76	736	156	786	76
637	79	687	85	737	139	787	82
638	69	688	77	738	75	788	69
639	77	689	76	739	75	789	69
640	74	690	178	740	88	790	79
641	76	691	158	741	75	791	122
642	69	692	176	742	76	792	82
643	86	693	161	743	83	793	78
644	75	694	135	744	73	794	72
645	78	695	79	745	144	795	74
646	72	696	135	746	120	796	72
647	74	697	73	747	77	797	165
648	74	698	152	748	142	798	79
649	83	699	144	749	70	799	77
650	87	700	80	750	70	800	78

(*Continued on p. 208*)

TABLE B.1   Continued

Record Number	Length	Record Number	Length	Record Number	Length	Record Number	Length
801	70	823	76	845	71	867	140
802	79	824	74	846	72	868	140
803	100	825	76	847	82	869	110
804	169	826	77	848	80	870	90
805	155	827	76	849	75	871	80
806	141	828	69	850	75	872	86
807	79	829	80	851	72	873	75
808	141	830	81	852	107	874	85
809	166	831	72	853	153	875	74
810	90	832	75	854	78	876	85
811	150	833	78	855	79	877	82
812	149	834	110	856	87	878	73
813	163	835	80	857	90	879	185
814	145	836	76	858	147	880	185
815	160	837	138	859	82	881	153
816	135	838	89	860	80	882	149
817	138	839	86	861	77	883	153
818	80	840	71	862	77	884	88
819	80	841	76	863	78	885	127
820	86	842	73	864	78	886	150
821	74	843	75	865	85	887	177
822	78	844	87	866	165	888	142

TABLE B.2   TOTAL LENGTH (IN MILLIMETERS) OF 854 MALE AND 797 FEMALE MOSQUITO FISH

Record Number	Males	Females	Record Number	Males	Females
1	19	34	51	24	28
2	17	30	52	22	28
3	21	30	53	23	28
4	20	28	54	24	33
5	18	31	55	22	34
6	21	28	56	23	32
7	20	35	57	24	36
8	18	35	58	20	44
9	21	28	59	20	34
10	17	27	60	22	33
11	17	34	61	22	35
12	21	27	62	24	37
13	18	30	63	31	32
14	23	56	64	22	34
15	24	52	65	23	50
16	20	49	66	28	45
17	21	37	67	19	34
18	22	30	68	22	32
19	22	35	69	21	37
20	18	34	70	23	35
21	23	47	71	22	37
22	16	34	72	24	37
23	24	33	73	20	37
24	20	33	74	23	34
25	16	32	75	17	40
26	21	33	76	22	40
27	17	32	77	24	38
28	16	31	78	20	33
29	24	32	79	20	30
30	24	35	80	23	30
31	27	38	81	20	31
32	22	35	82	18	30
33	21	36	83	21	33
34	21	34	84	25	35
35	23	32	85	22	51
36	24	33	86	29	32
37	22	35	87	19	31
38	21	34	88	22	37
39	23	34	89	21	30
40	22	37	90	20	34
41	22	35	91	20	35
42	22	32	92	23	33
43	22	33	93	22	35
44	22	35	94	18	33
45	28	31	95	22	30
46	22	34	96	21	40
47	22	30	97	22	37
48	24	31	98	21	36
49	21	30	99	22	32
50	22	32	100	24	30

(*Continued on p. 210*)

TABLE B.2   Continued

Record Number	Males	Females	Record Number	Males	Females
101	17	31	151	24	30
102	22	32	152	26	40
103	23	31	153	24	34
104	21	43	154	23	37
105	21	39	155	23	36
106	19	36	156	24	33
107	24	36	157	25	32
108	20	34	158	24	30
109	23	34	159	23	35
110	21	37	160	24	30
111	19	34	161	22	38
112	22	38	162	21	37
113	22	35	163	23	31
114	21	35	164	26	33
115	23	36	165	24	37
116	20	34	166	24	38
117	21	38	167	22	32
118	20	33	168	21	36
119	20	30	169	24	33
120	23	33	170	21	35
121	20	30	171	26	34
122	21	36	172	22	36
123	20	36	173	21	37
124	20	31	174	22	33
125	24	36	175	22	32
126	24	32	176	26	34
127	24	27	177	27	36
128	18	30	178	25	32
129	19	49	179	30	34
130	21	32	180	25	29
131	21	30	181	25	49
132	19	32	182	25	33
133	25	36	183	20	41
134	23	32	184	25	30
135	25	34	185	23	34
136	23	33	186	22	47
137	24	31	187	25	30
138	24	31	188	21	32
139	23	34	189	25	30
140	25	34	190	22	31
141	23	37	191	21	31
142	22	32	192	24	32
143	24	35	193	24	27
144	23	30	194	22	27
145	23	39	195	25	47
146	21	32	196	23	30
147	24	36	197	27	27
148	24	38	198	24	27
149	23	36	199	25	29
150	21	34	200	23	35

TABLE B.2   Continued

Record Number	Males	Females	Record Number	Males	Females
201	22	32	251	26	29
202	23	34	252	25	51
203	24	32	253	27	39
204	21	32	254	22	35
205	22	31	255	25	32
206	22	30	256	23	32
207	25	30	257	23	35
208	21	31	258	22	35
209	21	32	259	21	35
210	22	31	260	25	36
211	23	26	261	24	31
212	24	27	262	25	35
213	22	26	263	21	32
214	21	27	264	22	36
215	25	48	265	26	34
216	23	30	266	27	29
217	20	33	267	21	30
218	21	33	268	24	36
219	20	30	269	24	29
220	23	36	270	24	32
221	26	34	271	26	34
222	24	35	272	25	34
223	21	37	273	22	37
224	21	33	274	25	32
225	21	30	275	24	35
226	20	34	276	19	37
227	20	33	277	27	34
228	20	30	278	27	34
229	19	34	279	24	39
230	22	33	280	22	34
231	26	32	281	23	38
232	24	31	282	24	31
233	26	30	283	22	34
234	21	34	284	25	29
235	28	36	285	22	30
236	27	31	286	22	32
237	24	33	287	21	30
238	27	32	288	21	30
239	20	31	289	22	30
240	27	35	290	23	30
241	21	30	291	20	30
242	22	33	292	25	30
243	27	30	293	24	28
244	25	38	294	23	31
245	26	33	295	24	33
246	24	36	296	27	31
247	27	33	297	22	25
248	27	31	298	22	29
249	24	31	299	23	30
250	27	35	300	21	37

(*Continued on p. 212*)

TABLE B.2   Continued

Record Number	Males	Females	Record Number	Males	Females
301	24	31	351	22	25
302	22	38	352	26	25
303	25	43	353	21	27
304	25	52	354	22	24
305	21	53	355	26	24
306	21	50	356	22	24
307	24	45	357	24	23
308	21	53	358	21	44
309	23	50	359	21	31
310	21	37	360	23	46
311	24	36	361	21	33
312	20	37	362	24	30
313	21	38	363	21	37
314	25	37	364	21	46
315	23	39	365	20	46
316	21	36	366	20	31
317	22	37	367	22	31
318	22	32	368	24	46
319	22	36	369	23	33
320	25	39	370	23	34
321	23	34	371	19	33
322	24	36	372	23	48
323	27	35	373	23	37
324	27	32	374	22	35
325	23	36	375	24	45
326	23	32	376	21	51
327	20	35	377	23	43
328	24	32	378	23	41
329	23	31	379	22	30
330	20	28	380	23	39
331	22	30	381	20	45
332	26	29	382	29	47
333	26	34	383	24	39
334	25	33	384	24	41
335	23	31	385	25	45
336	21	27	386	25	31
337	22	29	387	22	30
338	21	31	388	25	33
339	20	30	389	24	45
340	20	28	390	22	30
341	23	38	391	22	39
342	23	37	392	24	29
343	20	32	393	21	30
344	24	35	394	23	36
345	25	33	395	22	40
346	23	32	396	21	42
347	26	30	397	19	31
348	21	31	398	22	30
349	20	27	399	22	29
350	23	27	400	24	28

TABLE B.2   Continued

Record Number	Males	Females	Record Number	Males	Females
401	23	31	451	23	29
402	24	35	452	22	29
403	28	29	453	24	28
404	22	30	454	20	28
405	24	27	455	21	28
406	21	25	456	23	27
407	20	29	457	21	29
408	24	26	458	25	25
409	24	28	459	21	29
410	23	28	460	21	28
411	23	34	461	22	28
412	22	35	462	23	27
413	22	32	463	25	29
414	21	33	464	22	24
415	21	34	465	23	25
416	22	40	466	23	24
417	20	30	467	21	28
418	21	35	468	25	27
419	24	35	469	25	25
420	29	27	470	24	28
421	26	30	471	25	27
422	27	34	472	23	27
423	23	29	473	23	24
424	26	32	474	22	28
425	25	34	475	20	50
426	24	31	476	21	37
427	27	31	477	24	42
428	25	29	478	19	37
429	28	30	479	22	46
430	23	31	480	23	37
431	30	30	481	22	44
432	30	31	482	24	51
433	24	32	483	24	37
434	23	31	484	19	51
435	26	30	485	20	40
436	26	30	486	24	36
437	23	31	487	24	33
438	23	44	488	21	43
439	20	31	489	22	32
440	22	34	490	22	46
441	22	30	491	23	33
442	24	30	492	25	39
443	21	30	493	22	40
444	20	30	494	20	43
445	25	25	495	20	37
446	24	26	496	24	43
447	23	23	497	20	44
448	30	26	498	23	33
449	23	24	499	22	38
450	29	28	500	21	38

(*Continued on p. 214*)

TABLE B.2   **Continued**

Record Number	Males	Females	Record Number	Males	Females
501	22	31	551	23	33
502	22	36	552	22	33
503	21	31	553	24	36
504	20	36	554	21	30
505	21	39	555	23	32
506	24	34	556	22	33
507	20	38	557	24	39
508	24	37	558	23	35
509	21	40	559	25	35
510	21	37	560	21	33
511	22	32	561	23	30
512	19	34	562	21	34
513	21	33	563	23	29
514	19	33	564	22	32
515	22	34	565	21	31
516	23	25	566	22	42
517	22	25	567	21	36
518	22	27	568	20	32
519	22	26	569	20	32
520	20	29	570	20	31
521	23	29	571	19	31
522	22	28	572	17	35
523	22	29	573	19	30
524	24	25	574	19	35
525	20	27	575	28	35
526	22	28	576	25	32
527	21	28	577	25	31
528	23	30	578	27	33
529	23	29	579	25	34
530	20	29	580	25	36
531	21	29	581	24	31
532	21	27	582	27	37
533	20	27	583	26	32
534	21	31	584	27	37
535	22	33	585	21	29
536	26	32	586	24	30
537	24	34	587	24	31
538	22	34	588	25	32
539	19	38	589	28	34
540	20	34	590	23	30
541	20	32	591	27	34
542	27	35	592	23	38
543	23	31	593	26	36
544	25	30	594	23	31
545	23	37	595	26	30
546	23	33	596	27	35
547	25	33	597	26	32
548	24	32	598	28	33
549	22	30	599	26	29
550	24	30	600	24	31

TABLE B.2   Continued

Record Number	Males	Females	Record Number	Males	Females
601	25	30	651	25	34
602	27	31	652	26	36
603	26	30	653	28	30
604	25	39	654	27	36
605	28	37	655	30	32
606	26	36	656	25	37
607	26	30	657	29	37
608	25	32	658	27	38
609	30	35	659	24	33
610	24	35	660	26	33
611	27	31	661	26	32
612	26	36	662	22	32
613	25	31	663	25	39
614	28	35	664	25	37
615	26	31	665	27	33
616	25	34	666	28	36
617	25	35	667	25	32
618	30	31	668	26	31
619	26	31	669	26	32
620	25	35	670	22	33
621	25	34	671	27	34
622	26	30	672	25	40
623	27	33	673	26	32
624	25	36	674	27	32
625	24	36	675	24	31
626	26	33	676	24	31
627	22	36	677	25	31
628	27	30	678	25	33
629	26	35	679	25	32
630	25	32	680	25	41
631	25	31	681	24	32
632	27	32	682	24	34
633	26	30	683	25	36
634	22	29	684	25	36
635	26	27	685	27	36
636	24	28	686	23	38
637	27	29	687	25	31
638	25	27	688	25	31
639	23	29	689	23	32
640	23	29	690	27	31
641	25	50	691	24	33
642	26	36	692	22	33
643	26	35	693	25	31
644	25	42	694	23	34
645	28	45	695	27	41
646	23	42	696	24	30
647	27	37	697	25	38
648	25	45	698	26	31
649	26	35	699	27	31
650	23	32	700	25	31

(*Continued on p. 216*)

TABLE B.2   Continued

Record Number	Males	Females	Record Number	Males	Females
701	23	30	751	26	41
702	26	33	752	30	40
703	22	31	753	24	41
704	25	33	754	31	45
705	24	30	755	23	32
706	27	29	756	25	41
707	25	47	757	26	39
708	26	47	758	30	40
709	23	48	759	24	42
710	25	50	760	24	41
711	25	42	761	25	39
712	24	44	762	23	39
713	25	44	763	24	41
714	25	34	764	25	42
715	26	43	765	28	41
716	26	45	766	25	40
717	26	45	767	26	39
718	24	41	768	24	40
719	25	40	769	25	44
720	26	44	770	25	40
721	28	47	771	27	43
722	25	49	772	25	38
723	23	47	773	26	40
724	24	37	774	23	34
725	25	43	775	26	36
726	25	40	776	24	34
727	26	38	777	27	33
728	26	32	778	24	35
729	27	41	779	28	41
730	23	45	780	26	44
731	23	42	781	26	37
732	27	40	782	23	37
733	23	37	783	23	34
734	27	42	784	22	37
735	24	44	785	25	37
736	24	43	786	24	40
737	24	40	787	23	43
738	25	34	788	25	38
739	24	40	789	24	42
740	24	45	790	27	33
741	27	39	791	23	32
742	30	47	792	23	31
743	24	36	793	26	32
744	24	38	794	26	31
745	30	44	795	27	30
746	26	34	796	27	28
747	26	36	797	28	29
748	23	48	798	26	
749	24	43	799	23	
750	28	42	800	22	

TABLE B.2   **Continued**

Record Number	Males	Females	Record Number	Males	Females
801	29		828	26	
802	27		829	28	
803	25		830	25	
804	25		831	26	
805	21		832	27	
806	26		833	25	
807	23		834	28	
808	26		835	28	
809	23		836	28	
810	31		837	26	
811	32		838	26	
812	32		839	27	
813	25		840	29	
814	27		841	28	
815	29		842	28	
816	30		843	27	
817	27		844	27	
818	26		845	28	
819	26		846	27	
820	29		847	23	
821	30		848	26	
822	24		849	27	
823	25		850	29	
824	26		851	24	
825	28		852	27	
826	27		853	27	
827	32		854	26	

TABLE B.3 SOME BEHAVIORAL AND PHYSICAL ATTRIBUTES OF A SAMPLE OF 165 UNIVERSITY STUDENTS
(Data obtained from a questionnaire and from measurements; names of the variables and the response codes are found at the end of the table*)

Record Number	Age	Sex	Aer	Wts	Smk	Caf	Jck	Pr	Rct
1	20	1	1	1	2	1	1	72	125
2	18	1	2	2	2	2	2	80	150
3	21	1	1	1	2	2	1	60	100
4	18	1	2	2	2	2	2	60	160
5	18	1	1	1	2	2	1	53	150
6	18	1	1	2	2	2	1	81	140
7	18	1	2	2	2	2	2	67	170
8	20	1	2	2	1	2	2	63	150
9	18	1	2	2	2	2	2	72	210
10	19	1	2	2	2	2	2	72	250
11	18	1	2	2	1	2	1	76	275
12	21	1	2	2	2	2	2	76	150
13	21	1	1	2	2	2	2	80	100
14	19	1	1	1	2	2	2	60	190
15	19	1	2	1	2	1	1	72	160
16	20	1	2	1	2	2	2	80	210
17	18	1	2	1	2	2	1	80	200
18	20	1	2	2	2	2	2	80	175
19	18	1	2	1	2	2	2	104	180
20	18	1	1	1	2	2	1	80	175
21	19	1	1	1	1	2	1	56	160
22	18	1	2	2	2	1	2	68	159
23	20	1	1	2	2	2	2	70	180
24	18	1	2	2	2	2	1	72	190
25	19	1	2	2	1	2	1	68	180
26	20	1	1	2	2	2	2	80	175
27	19	1	2	1	2	2	1	78	150
28	18	1	2	1	2	2	1	62	200
29	18	1	2	2	2	2	1	64	200
30	18	1	2	1	2	2	1	88	197
31	20	1	2	2	2	2	2	65	200
32	18	1	2	1	2	1	2	68	175
33	23	1	2	1	2	2	2	73	140
34	18	1	2	1	1	2	1	60	155
35	18	1	2	2	2	2	2	96	180
36	18	1	2	1	2	2	1	78	210
37	18	1	2	2	1	1	2	92	170
38	18	1	2	2	2	2	2	100	105
39	21	1	1	1	2	2	2	80	175
40	17	1	1	2	2	2	1	76	180
41	20	1	2	2	2	2	2	71	203
42	18	1	2	2	1	1	1	77	193
43	19	1	2	1	2	2	2	70	133
44	18	1	2	2	1	1	1	85	190
45	18	1	2	2	2	1	1	80	153
46	21	1	2	2	2	2	2	68	150
47	19	1	1	2	2	2	1	76	168

TABLE B.3   **Continued**

Record Number	Age	Sex	Aer	Wts	Smk	Caf	Jck	Pr	Rct
48	18	1	2	1	2	2	1	84	183
49	23	1	2	1	1	2	1	84	183
50	22	1	2	2	2	2	2	72	150
51	19	1	1	1	2	1	1	60	190
52	19	1	2	1	2	1	1	68	150
53	19	1	1	1	2	2	1	68	183
54	18	1	1	1	2	2	1	66	137
55	18	1	2	1	2	1	2	63	145
56	19	1	1	2	2	2	1	78	180
57	18	1	2	2	2	2	1	74	110
58	18	1	1	1	2	1	1	68	187
59	19	1	1	1	1	2	1	72	186
60	18	1	1	2	2	1	1	75	223
61	18	1	2	2	2	1	2	80	176
62	18	1	2	2	1	2	1	84	180
63	19	1	1	1	2	2	1	56	100
64	19	1	1	1	2	2	1	56	100
65	19	1	1	1	2	2	1	80	146
66	18	1	2	2	2	2	2	76	190
67	18	1	2	1	2	1	2	80	175
68	18	1	2	2	1	1	2	90	170
69	18	1	2	2	2	1	1	88	130
70	18	1	2	1	2	1	2	86	186
71	19	1	2	1	1	1	2	76	243
72	23	1	2	1	2	2	1	84	190
73	20	1	2	1	2	1	2	82	180
74	21	1	2	2	1	1	2	90	166
75	19	1	2	2	2	2	1	68	210
76	19	1	1	2	2	1	1	69	170
77	18	1	1	1	2	2	1	68	156
78	18	2	1	1	2	2	1	80	110
79	18	2	1	1	2	1	1	92	170
80	18	2	2	2	2	2	2	82	205
81	18	2	2	2	1	2	2	80	180
82	21	2	2	2	2	1	2	76	163
83	18	2	2	2	2	1	1	80	140
84	20	2	2	2	2	2	2	88	166
85	18	2	1	1	2	2	1	80	150
86	18	2	1	2	2	2	2	80	150
87	18	2	2	2	1	1	1	82	120
88	18	2	1	1	2	2	1	80	70
89	18	2	2	2	2	2	1	94	150
90	18	2	2	2	2	2	2	93	150
91	18	2	2	2	1	1	1	84	180
92	18	2	2	2	2	2	1	72	100
93	18	2	2	2	2	2	2	86	150
94	18	2	2	2	2	2	2	80	190
95	18	2	2	2	2	2	1	74	100
96	18	2	2	1	2	2	2	73	210
97	18	2	2	2	2	2	1	81	220

(*Continued on p. 220*)

TABLE B.3   Continued

Record Number	Age	Sex	Aer	Wts	Smk	Caf	Jck	Pr	Rct
98	19	2	2	2	1	2	2	72	225
99	18	2	2	2	1	1	2	80	200
100	18	2	2	1	2	2	2	76	275
101	18	2	2	2	2	1	2	80	250
102	18	2	1	2	2	2	1	80	270
103	19	2	1	2	2	2	2	89	240
104	18	2	2	2	2	2	2	94	150
105	21	2	1	2	2	2	1	64	155
106	19	2	2	2	2	2	1	76	135
107	19	2	2	2	2	2	2	59	240
108	19	2	1	2	1	2	1	140	260
109	18	2	2	2	1	2	1	79	110
110	18	2	2	2	2	2	2	63	180
111	21	2	2	2	2	2	2	80	190
112	17	2	2	2	2	2	2	88	310
113	23	2	1	1	2	1	1	72	160
114	18	2	2	2	2	2	2	80	190
115	18	2	2	2	2	1	2	82	212
116	17	2	2	2	2	1	2	104	235
117	18	2	2	2	2	2	2	80	220
118	19	2	1	2	2	1	2	72	200
119	18	2	2	2	2	2	1	89	163
120	18	2	2	2	2	2	1	82	180
121	18	2	2	1	2	1	1	89	230
122	18	2	2	2	1	1	1	86	200
123	19	2	2	2	2	2	1	80	130
124	19	2	1	1	2	1	2	70	173
125	18	2	2	2	2	1	1	93	208
126	18	2	2	2	1	2	2	75	200
127	19	2	2	2	2	2	2	86	250
128	18	2	1	2	2	1	2	84	150
129	19	2	1	2	2	2	2	88	196
130	19	2	2	2	2	1	2	106	126
131	20	2	1	1	2	1	2	65	176
132	18	2	1	1	2	2	1	68	206
133	20	2	1	2	2	2	2	80	177
134	18	2	2	2	2	1	1	102	181
135	24	2	2	2	2	2	2	120	136
136	18	2	2	2	1	1	2	88	163
137	18	2	2	2	2	2	1	91	175
138	18	2	2	2	2	1	1	66	167
139	19	2	1	2	2	2	2	85	156
140	18	2	1	2	2	2	1	43	213
141	19	2	1	1	2	2	1	70	228
142	18	2	2	2	2	2	1	84	243
143	37	2	2	2	1	1	2	80	225
144	18	2	2	2	2	1	2	72	200
145	19	2	1	2	2	2	2	126	163
146	19	2	1	1	2	1	2	92	225
147	38	2	2	2	2	1	2	85	241

TABLE B.3 Continued

Record Number	Age	Sex	Aer	Wts	Smk	Caf	Jck	Pr	Rct
148	18	2	1	2	2	1	2	76	130
149	28	2	1	2	2	2	2	108	207
150	18	2	2	2	2	1	2	107	255
151	18	2	2	2	2	2	1	76	223
152	18	2	1	1	2	2	1	64	150
153	18	2	2	2	2	2	2	88	190
154	18	2	2	2	2	2	1	80	160
155	18	2	1	1	2	1	2	64	183
156	18	2	2	2	2	2	1	88	166
157	20	2	2	2	2	1	2	84	172
158	18	2	1	2	2	2	1	65	152
159	18	2	1	1	2	2	1	63	250
160	18	2	1	1	2	2	1	63	250
161	18	2	2	2	2	1	2	84	250
162	19	2	1	2	2	1	2	80	200
163	24	2	1	1	2	2	2	120	200
164	23	2	2	2	2	2	2	101	210
165	18	2	2	2	2	2	1	66	170

*Variables and codes. Sex: 1 = male, 2 = female
Aer: Response to the question "Do you do aerobic exercise on a regular basis?"
   1 = yes, 2 = no
Wts: Response to the question "Do you work out with weights on a regular basis?"
   1 = yes, 2 = no
Smk: Response to the question "Do you smoke?" 1 = yes, 2 = no
Caf: Response to the question "Have you consumed caffeine in the past 2 hours?"
   1 = yes, 2 = no
Jck: Response to the question "Have you participated in a varsity sport within the past
   year?" 1 = yes, 2 = no
Pr: Pulse rate in beats per minute
Rct: Reaction time in milliseconds

Answers to Exercises for Chapters 3 through 9

Slight discrepancies between these answers and your answers are to be expected because of differences in the number of significant digits used in calculating and/or because of rounding errors.

CHAPTER 3

3.1

Mean 6.00
Median 6.50
Range 1–11
Sum of Squares 260.00
Variance 8.9655
Standard Deviation 2.9942

3.2

Mean 30.3846
Median 23.00
Range 12–56
Sum of Squares 3137.0769
Variance 261.4231
Standard Deviation 16.1686

3.3

Mean 53.9643
Median 59.5
Range 9–98
Sum of Squares 19332.9640
Variance 716.0357
Standard Deviation 26.7588

3.4

Mean 55.6976
Median 56.5
Range 47.0–62.4
Sum of Squares 755.6698
Variance 18.4310
Standard Deviation 4.2931

3.5

Mean 181.8176
Median 181.5
Range 161–202
Sum of Squares 63680743
Variance 43.3202
Standard Deviation 6.5818

3.6

Mean 274.2100
Median 295.5
Range 66–456
Sum of Squares 867554.59
Variance 8763.1777
Standard Deviation 93.6118

3.12

Median = 2

3.13

299 pits in 100 quadrates; mean = 2.99 pits/quadrate

3.14

770 larvae in 197 leaves; mean = 3.9086 larvae/leaf

3.15

Mean 120.0338
Variance 1759.6742
Standard Deviation 41.9485
n 888

3.16

Mean 23.598
Variance 6.964
Standard Deviation 2.639
n 854

3.17

Mean 34.292
Variance 30.217
Standard Deviation 5.497
n 797

3.18

Mean 78.81
Variance 182.52
Standard Deviation 13.51
n 165

3.19

Mean 179.67
Variance 1634.58
Standard Deviation 40.43
n 165

CHAPTER 4

4.1

0.25

4.2

0.25

4.3

0.50

4.4

0.23

4.5

0.3437

4.6

0.0321

4.7

0.3302

4.8

0.9042

4.9

0.3125

4.10

0.3437

4.11

0.0156

4.12

0.0156

4.13

0.1780

4.14

0.1318

4.15

0.9624

4.16

0.00024

4.18

$p = 0.0007979$,
$F =$ approximately 1 family (0.7979)

4.19

0.9379

4.20

0.1560

4.21

0.2456

4.22

0.0012

4.24

x	p(x)	f(x)
0	0.0503	5.03
1	0.1504	15.04
2	0.2248	22.48
3	0.2240	22.40
4	0.1675	16.75
5	0.1001	10.01
6	0.0499	4.99
7	0.0213	2.13
8	0.0080	0.80

4.26

0.0000536

4.27

0.0117

4.28

x	p(x)	f(x)
0	0.0201	3.96
1	0.0784	15.44
2	0.1533	30.20
3	0.1997	39.34
4	0.1952	38.45
5	0.1526	30.06
6	0.0994	19.58
7	0.0555	10.93
8	0.0271	5.34

4.30

0.0271

4.31

0.0459

4.32

$\mu = 1.6667$ phage/cell; $p(0) = 0.1889$; $p(5) = 0.0202$

4.33

$\mu = 0.6$ phage/cell; $p (\geq 3) = 0.0231$

4.34

$\mu = 1.6667$

x	p(x)
0	0.1889
1	0.3148
2	0.2623
3	0.1457
4	0.0607
5	0.0202

4.35

$\mu = 0.6$

x	p(x)
0	0.5488
1	0.3293
2	0.0988
3	0.0198
4	0.0030
5	0.0004

4.36
0.0021

4.37
0.0455

4.38
0.6331

4.39
23.52 to 45.05

4.40
0.1814

4.41
0.1292

4.42
0.2386

4.43
113.63 to 190.55

4.44
0.0968

4.45
0.00001

4.46
0.3707

4.47
0.0021

4.48
0.8060

4.49
0.9723

CHAPTER 5

5.8
90%; 181.81 ± 0.895
95%; 181.81 ± 1.069
99%; 181.81 ± 1.413

5.9
90%; 274.21 ± 15.519
95%; 274.21 ± 18.533
99%; 274.21 ± 24.583

5.10
90%; 55.698 ± 1.116
95%; 55.698 ± 1.339
99%; 55.698 ± 1.791

5.11
90%; 19.2556 ± 1.5895
95%; 19.2556 ± 1.9707
99%; 19.2556 ± 2.8672

5.12
90%; 364.2500 ± 56.5054
95%; 364.2500 ± 69.2514
99%; 364.2500 ± 97.7205

5.13
90%; 45.1818 ± 5.4473
95%; 45.1818 ± 6.6967
99%; 45.1818 ± 9.5252

5.14
90%; 35.4000 ± 2.8489
95%; 35.4000 ± 3.4698
99%; 35.4000 ± 4.8159

5.15
90%; 4.9760 ± 0.2877
95%; 4.9760 ± 0.3471
99%; 4.9760 ± 0.4703

5.16
90%; 1934.6429 ± 247.9211
95%; 1934.6429 ± 302.4399
99%; 1934.6429 ± 421.7023

5.17
H_0: $\mu \leq 10$ ppb
H_1: $\mu > 10$ ppb
$t = 2.500$

5.18
H_0: $\mu \geq 50$ H_1: $\mu < 50$
$t = -2.8947$

5.19
H_0: $\mu = 100$ H_1: $\mu <> 100$
$t = 5.367$

CHAPTER 6

6.1
H_0: μ(men) $=$ μ(women)
H_1: μ(men) $<>$ μ(women)
$t = -3.83$

6.2
H_0: μ(men) $=$ μ(women)
H_1: μ(men) $<>$ μ(women)
$t = -1.57$

6.3
H_0: μ(largemouth) $=$ μ(smallmouth)
H_1: μ(largemouth) $<>$ μ(smallmouth)
$t = 11.33$

6.4
H_0: μ(A) $\leq$ μ(B)
H_1: μ(A) $>$ μ(B)
$t = 0.95$

6.5
H_0: μ(down) $\leq$ μ(up)
H_1: μ(down) $>$ μ(up)
$t = 5.14$

6.6
H_0: μ(exposed) $\geq$ μ(untreated)
H_1: μ(exposed) $<$ μ(untreated)
$t = 5.3780$

6.7
H_0: μ(A) $=$ μ(B)
H_1: μ(A) $<>$ μ(B)
$t = 0.5548$

6.8
H_0: μ(infected) $\leq$ μ(healthy)
H_1: μ(infected) $>$ μ(healthy)
$t = 3.7149$

6.9
H_0: μ(glucose) $=$ μ(sucrose)
H_1: μ(glucose) $<>$ μ(sucrose)
$t = 0.7310$

6.10
H_0: μ(treated) $\leq$ μ(control)
H_1: μ(treated) $>$ μ(control)
$t = 2.671$

6.11
H_0: μ(with) $\leq$ μ(without)
H_1: μ(with) $>$ μ(without)
$t = 6.1612$

6.12
H_0: μ(A) $=$ μ(B)
H_1: μ(A) $<>$ μ(B)
$t = 2.9414$

6.13
H_0: μ(coniferous) $=$ μ(deciduous)
H_1: μ(coniferous) $<>$ μ(deciduous)
$t = 4.1210$

6.14
H_0: μ(athletes) $\leq$ μ(non)
H_1: μ(athletes) $>$ μ(non)
$t = -0.25$

6.15
H_0: μ(smokers) $\leq$ μ(non)
H_1: μ(smokers) $>$ μ(non)
$t = -0.67$

6.17
$U = 8.5$

6.18
$U = 5$

6.19
$U = 32.5$

6.20
$U = 4$

6.21
$U = 39.5$

6.22
$U = 34$

6.23
H_0: μ(post $-$ pre) ≤ 0
H_1: μ(post $-$ pre) > 0
$t = 10.6215$

6.24
H_0: μ(difference) $= 0$
H_1: μ(difference) $<> 0$
$t = 4.27$

6.25
H_0: μ(difference) $= 0$
H_1: μ(difference) $<> 0$
$t = 2.1394$

6.26
H_0: μ(difference) $= 0$
H_1: μ(difference) $<> 0$
$t = 2.9351$

6.27
H_0: μ(wall $-$ center) ≤ 0
H_1: μ(wall $-$ center) > 0
$t = 2.3904$

6.28
$T = 2.5$

6.29
$T = 0$

6.30
$T = 13.5$

6.31
$p = 0.0899$

6.32
$p = 0.06$

6.33
$p = 0.029$

6.34
$p = 0.1$

CHAPTER 7

7.1

Source	Sum of Squares	df	MS	F
Between-Groups	6.2713	2	3.1356	30.87
Error	1.2191	12	0.1016	
Total	7.4904	14		

7.2

Source	Sum of Squares	df	MS	F
Between-Groups	0.09695	2	0.0485	89.81
Error	0.00814	15	0.00054	
Total	0.1051	17		

7.3

Source	Sum of Squares	df	MS	F
Between-Groups	632.95	3	210.98	70.33
Error	48.00	16	3.00	
Total	680.95	19		

7.4

Source	Sum of Squares	df	MS	F
Between-Groups	2365.6	4	591.4	21.05
Error	983.5	35	28.1	
Total	3349.1	39		

7.5

Source	Sum of Squares	df	MS	F
Between-Groups	1740.4	2	870.2	79.11
Error	132.0	12	11.0	
Total	1872.4	14		

7.6

Source	Sum of Squares	df	MS	F
Between-Groups	2112.47	2	1256.23	10.95
Error	3097.00	27	114.70	
Total	5609.47	29		

7.7

Source	Sum of Squares	df	MS	F
Between-Groups	3785.65	4	946.41	72.78
Error	455.13	35	13.00	
Total	4240.78	39		

7.8

Source	Sum of Squares	df	MS	F
Between-Groups	45.31	2	22.65	5.81
Error	89.65	23	3.9	
Total	134.96	25		

7.9

Source	Sum of Squares	df	MS	F
Between-Groups	145.6389	3	48.5463	19.64
Error	79.1111	32	2.4722	
Total	224.7500	35		

7.10

Source	Sum of Squares	df	MS	F
Between-Groups	1442.1333	2	721.0667	16.06
Error	538.8000	12	44.9000	
Total	1980.9333	14		

7.11

Source	Sum of Squares	df	MS	F
Between-Groups	3169.44	2	1584.72	15.63
Blocks	15573.61	5	3114.72	
Error	1013.89	10	101.39	
Total	19756.94	17		

7.12

Source	Sum of Squares	df	MS	F
Between-Groups	1049.20	2	524.60	24.10
Blocks	523.07	4	130.77	
Error	174.13	8	21.77	
Total	1746.40	14		

7.13

Source	Sum of Squares	df	MS	F
Between-Groups	1044.40	2	522.20	14.16
Blocks	39876.27	4	9969.07	
Error	294.93	8	36.87	
Total	41215.60	14		

7.14

Source	Sum of Squares	df	MS	F
Between-Groups	7704.93	2	3852.47	60.54
Blocks	24308.93	4	6077.23	
Error	509.07	8	63.63	
Total	32522.93	14		

7.15

Source	Sum of Squares	df	MS	F
Between-Groups	95033.83	3	31677.94	27.71
Blocks	2460.83	5	492.17	
Error	17149.17	15	1143.28	
Total	114643.83	23		

7.16

Source	Sum of Squares	df	MS	F
Between-Groups	587.56	2	293.78	29.05
Blocks	389.56	2	194.78	
Error	40.44	4	10.11	
Total	1017.56	8		

7.17

Source	Sum of Squares	df	MS	F
Between-Groups	18851.44	2	9425.72	1025.8
Blocks	5013.78	5	1002.76	
Error	91.89	10	9.19	
Total	23957.11	17		

7.18

Source	Sum of Squares	df	MS	F
Between-Groups	178188.50	2	89094.25	17.63
Blocks	84247.00	3	28082.33	
Error	30321.50	6	5053.58	
Total	292757.00	11		

7.19

Source	Sum of Squares	df	MS	F
Between-Groups	3592.56	4	898.14	16.08
Blocks	3439.76	4	859.94	
Error	893.44	16	55.84	
Total	7925.76	24		

7.20

Source	Sum of Squares	df	MS	F
Between-Groups	483.44	2	241.72	110.43
Blocks	1369.11	5	273.82	
Error	21.89	10	2.19	
Total	1874.44	17		

7.21

Source	Sum of Squares	df	MS	F
Strain	19683.63	2	9841.81	33.3
Treatment	58569.85	2	29284.93	99.07
Interaction	407.23	4	101.81	0.34
Error	5320.67	18	295.59	
Total	83981.41	26		

7.22

Source	Sum of Squares	df	MS	F
Sex	473126	2	236563	1442
Stress	16864	2	8432	51.41
Interaction	4401	4	1100	6.71
Error	7389	45	164	
Total	501780	53		

7.23

Source	Sum of Squares	df	MS	F
Temperature	1059.73	2	529.87	21.3
Feedings	1365.73	2	682.87	27.4
Interaction	50.13	4	12.53	0.5
Error	896.40	36	24.90	
Total	3372.00	44		

7.24

Source	Sum of Squares	df	MS	F
Age	6661.67	2	3330.83	46.9
Sex	616.53	1	616.53	8.68
Interaction	622.07	2	311.03	4.38
Error	1704.40	24	71.02	
Total	9604.67	29		

Exercises 7.25 and 7.26 are unbalanced factorial designs and are best done by computer. If using MINITAB, use the GLM option.

7.27
$\chi^2 = 0.1751$

7.28
$\chi^2 = 0.8019$

7.29
$\chi^2 = 2.2657$

7.30
$\chi^2 = 1.0297$

7.31
$\chi^2 = 1.1930$

7.32
$\chi^2 = 2.0551$

7.33
$\chi^2 = 7.5256$

7.34
$\chi^2 = 47.8193$

7.35
$H = 9.39$

7.36
$H = 18.12$

7.37
$H = 12.42$

7.38
$H = 10.81$

7.39
$H = 10.38$

7.40
$H = 21.13$

7.41
$\chi^2 = 22.1$

7.42
$\chi^2 = 11.85$

7.43
$\chi^2 = 9.33$

7.44
$\chi^2 = 6.00$

7.45
$\chi^2 = 11.75$

7.46
$\chi^2 = 12.00$

CHAPTER 8

8.1
$r = 0.827$

8.2
$r = 0.695$

8.3
$r = 0.590$

8.4
$r = 0.590$

8.5
$r = 0.747$

8.6
$r = 0.373$

8.7
$r = 0.994$

8.8
$r = -0.049$

8.9
$r = 0.141$

8.10
$r = 0.449$

8.11
$r = 0.628$

8.12
$r = 0.617$

8.13
$r = 0.221$

8.14
$r = 0.134$

8.15
$\hat{y} = -1.90 + 10.7x; r^2 = 0.999$

Source	SS	df	MS	F
Regression	33093	1	33093	4750.44
Error	28	4	7	
Total	33121	5		

8.16
$\hat{y} = 75.5 - 8.25x; r^2 = 0.59$
 (requires log transformation of
 both variables)

Source	SS	df	MS	F
Regression	3456.4	1	3456.4	5.73
Error	2414.4	4	603.6	
Total	5870.8	5		

8.17

$\hat{y} = 100 + 3.90x$; $r^2 = 0.909$

Source	SS	df	MS	F
Regression	912.60	1	912.60	70.23
Error	90.96	7	12.99	
Total	1003.56	8		

8.18

$\hat{y} = 0.983 + 0.519x$; $r^2 = 0.997$

Source	SS	df	MS	F
Regression	4.7112	1	4.7112	1179.49
Error	0.0160	4	0.0040	
Total	4.7272	5		

8.19

$\hat{y} = 0.00257 + 0.00134x$; $r^2 = 0.978$
($y = 1$/rate, $x = 1$ substrate concentration)

Source	SS	df	MS	F
Regression	0.0000164	1	0.0000164	134.29
Error	0.00000037	3	0.00000012	
Total	0.00001677	4		

8.20

$\hat{y} = -122 + 71.2x$; $r^2 = 0.759$

Source	SS	df	MS	F
Regression	152140	1	152140	41.01
Error	48227	13	3710	
Total	200367	14		

8.21

$\hat{y} = 15.1 + 1.46x$; $r^2 = 0.932$

Source	SS	df	MS	F
Regression	235.65	1	235.65	124.16
Error	17.08	9	1.90	
Total	252.73	10		

8.22

$\hat{y} = 0.103 + 0.0276x$; $r^2 = 0.491$

Source	SS	df	MS	F
Regression	1.0687	1	1.0687	26.96
Error	1.1099	28	0.0396	
Total	2.1786	29		

8.23

$\hat{y} = 6.99 - 0.675x$; $r^2 = 0.974$

Source	SS	df	MS	F
Regression	114.32	1	114.32	698.74
Error	3.11	19	0.16	
Total	117.43	20		

8.24

$\hat{y} = 6.52 + 0.811x$; $r^2 = 0.909$

Source	SS	df	MS	F
Regression	2137.0	1	2137.0	240.1
Error	213.6	24	8.9	
Total	2350.6	25		

CHAPTER 9

9.1

$\chi^2 = 25$

9.2

$\chi^2 = 0.16$

9.3

$\chi^2 = 0.333$

9.4

$\chi^2 = 0.1004$

9.5

$\chi^2 = 0.1500$

9.6

$\chi^2 = 2.55$

9.7

$\chi^2 = 0.2667$

9.8

$\chi^2 = 1.67$

9.9

$\chi^2 = 1.33$

Exercises 9.10 through 9.13 are intended to be done by computer.

9.14

$\chi^2 = 30.29$ (The first 2 categories should be combined, as should the last 2 categories. This gives 4 degrees of freedom.)

9.15

$\chi^2 = 1.7124$

9.16

$\chi^2 = 26.7561$ (The first 4 categories should be combined, giving 2 degrees of freedom.)

9.17

$\chi^2 = 32.06$

9.18

$\chi^2 = 18.8621$ (The last 2 categories should be combined, giving 4 degrees of freedom.)

9.19

$\chi^2 = 0.2023$ (The last 3 categories should be combined, giving 6 degrees of freedom.)

9.20

$\chi^2 = 50.89$ (The first 2 and last 2 categories should be combined, giving 8 degrees of freedom.)

9.21

$\chi^2 = 39.40$

9.22

$\chi^2 = 12.04$

9.23

$\chi^2 = 10.38$

9.24

$\chi^2 = 24.2$

Exercises 9.25 through 9.28 are intended to be done by computer.

9.29

$\chi^2 = 57.53$

9.30

$p = 0.0513$ (one-tailed)

9.31

$p < 7 \times 10^{-11}$

9.32

$p < 10^{-6}$

Index

A

Addition rule, 38
Alpha risk, 78
Alternative hypothesis, 73
Analysis of variance (ANOVA)
  assumptions of, 108–109, 130
  completely randomized design,
    109–118
  computer-generated, 135, 136
  explanation of, 106
  and factorial resign, 123–130
  nonparametric alternatives to,
    131–135
  and randomized complete
    blocks design, 118–122
  rationale of, 106–108
  transformations in, 130–131
Arcsine transformation, 131
Arithmetic mean. *See* Mean
Attributes, 8–9
Average. *See* Mean

B

Bar graphs. *See also* Histograms
  description of, 12
  for discrete variables, 16
  illustration of, 13
Bartlett's chi-square test for
  homogeneity of variances,
  128–129
Beta risk, 78
Between-groups variance, 107
Binomial distributions
  calculation of, 40–41
  examples of, 37–39, 41–43
  explanation of, 37
  normal approximation of,
    55–57
  properties of, 37

C

Central limit theorem, 65
Central tendency, 24–25
Chi-square distribution
  critical values of, 198
  explanation of, 128
  illustration of, 129
Chi-square goodness of fit test,
  182–187
Classificatory scale, 9
Coefficient of determination,
  167–168
Completely random design ANOVA
  with fixed effects (model I),
    110, 116–117, 152
  with random effects (model II),
    117–118, 152
Computer programs
  graphing capabilities of, 16, 17
  inferences concerning two
    populations performed by,
    95
  linear regression using, 170,
    171
  summary statistics for sample
    variable given by, 29
Confidence intervals
  for β, 167
  cautions regarding, 69
  explanation of, 68, 70
  of group means, 115
  when population standard
    deviation (σ) is known,
    68–69
  when population standard
    deviation (σ) is unknown,
    69–70

D

Data, 8, 9
Degrees of freedom, 28
Dependent variable, 152
Derived variable, 9
Discrete probability distributions
  binomial distribution as, 36–43
  Poisson distribution as, 43–46

Continuous variables
  explanation of, 8
  frequency distributions of,
    12–16
  value assumed by, 14
Correlation analysis
  nonparametric, 159–160
  regression vs., 152–155, 160
  uses of, 152
Correlation coefficient
  explanation of, 156
  Pearson, 156–158, 201
  r as sample, 156
  square of, 168
Critical values
  of chi-square distribution, 183,
    198
  explanation of, 75
  of F distribution, 200
  of Pearson correlation
    coefficient, 158, 201
  of Spearman rank correlation
    coefficient, 202
  of t distribution, 197
  for Tukey test, 201
  of U for Mann-Whitney test,
    199
  of Wilcoxon test, 199
Cumulative frequency distributions
  computation of, 53, 55
  explanation of, 52–53
  illustration of, 54

D

Discrete variables
  explanation of, 8
  frequency distributions of,
    11–13
  graphs of, 16
  normal distributions and,
    57–58
  value assumed by, 14
Dispersion measures, 25–27
Distribution-free methods, 58. *See
  also* Nonparametric tests

E

Error variance
  in ANOVA, 127
  explanation of, 90, 106
  kept at minimum, 110
  testing for equality of, 128
Estimated regression line, 162, 165
Estimation, 64–67
Expected distributions, 44, 45
Experimental data, 116–117
Extrapolation, 168

F

F distribution
  critical values of, 200
  explanation of, 107
  illustration of, 108
Factorial design
  ANOVA, 123–127
  explanation of, 123
  with more than two levels of
    one of main effects, 127
Fisher exact probability test,
  187–188
Fixed effects, 110
Frequency distributions
  computer-generated graphic
    representations of, 16, 17
  of continuous variables, 12–16